Heartatude

The 9 Principles of Heart-Centered Success

by

ALISOUN MACKENZIE

G2P Publishing

Published in 2015 by G2P Publishing

ISBN Paperback: 978-0-9930752-0-9
ISBN eBook: 978-0-9930752-1-6

This book was produced with the help of
Indie Authors World.

Cover design by Deanna Everett

Praise for Heartatude

One of the many unique qualities of Heartatude is its authenticity. Alisoun Mackenzie didn't simply sit in her office and come up with a theory about how to both live life and create business with heart. This book comes from a deep experience of applying the principles within it in a variety of situations, and from within the trenches of real life. This is a manual for heartful living that will create deep growth for the reader on a variety of levels. Highly recommended.

Sasha Allenby, co-author of *Matrix Reimprinting Using EFT* & author of *Write an Evolutionary Self-Help Book*

In a world of technological advancements Heartatude brings us back to the core values of humanity. Its emphasis on self nurture to engender success is a key element that has been neglected in today' s turgid lifestyles. The book draws from a wide range of cultural belief systems backed up by science where relevant. This is a valuable toolkit that will enable us to move towards more symbiotic relationships and thus fulfilment.

Dr Y Chan, general practitioner

Times are changing. The survival of the fittest approach to success is becoming extinct as a more heart-centered approach emerges. One that not only brings inner contentment and happiness to those who embrace it, but that also makes a difference to others, too. This book will inspire you to do just that – enjoy the journey!

Lorraine Murray, author of *Calm Kids* and owner of Feel Good Therapies

I LOVE this book; it connected with me at a deep level. Alisoun writes from her heart, sharing stories and ideas that inspire and engage not only the head but the heart and soul. The authenticity of her words offers practical ways to tackle life's challenges and achieve real transformation. It is also an easy book to read, it has all the elements that I love – science, rational explanations, energy, fun, optimism, hope, and the important part: how to make it work for you. It's all here and more – if you want to create change in your life, have more happiness and success, then buy this book. Read it, absorb it, act on it, and be grateful that you found it.

Kim Macleod, author of *From Heartbreak to Happiness* & owner of Indie Authors World

We are living in a time of tangible change, and many are looking for ways to support the shift in our collective consciousness. Heartatude provides an opportunity to examine, not only what you want to achieve in terms of your own success and happiness, but also a way to do this in full alignment with your values and integrity. Embody the change within, and create it in the world around you!
Jennifer Main, theta healing instructor & author

Alisoun embodies the very principles of Heartatude, not just by her words but her actions. This book will help you to get clear on what success means to you, and inspire you to make that vision a reality.
Cindy Schulson, authentic marketing expert

This book is testament to a life dreamed and a life lived in the fullness of *Carpe Diem*. I was gripped from the first page and know it will be a reference that I will go back to time and again as its leading life principles are authentic, meaningful, and can have a dramatically positive impact on your life. If this book finds you – you were meant to have it as part of your life journey. I relish every page.
Bonnie Clarke, recruitment company director

Heartatude will give you simple and practical techniques as well as a wonderful feeling of warmth whenever you finish a chapter.
Jill Cruikshank, coaching & development consultant

Heartatude is a must read for anyone searching for the missing link and who knows there's another way to live or do business. It will help you know who you really are, encourage you to do the work you love, convince you that you deserve to earn good money doing just that, and still be of service to the planet; all in a heart-centred way. An easy-to-read book packed with inspiration, practical hints and tips – what a joy to read!
Jo Turner, meditation teacher & holistic practitioner

Uplifting, illuminating, and enlightening, Heartatude is a profoundly simple concept that offersyou an authenticand compassionate approach for successand abetter world. I highly recommend this book. My heart was swollen with possibilities just reading these pages.
Deborah L. Hall, author of *Million Dollar Moments*

What a terrific book - thought provoking, engaging and inspiring! Heartatude takes you on a voyage of discovery. Believe me if you think you know about this subject think again, you will learn so many new wonderful ideas.

Glenda Barton, happy and guilt free mum

Alisoun is an inspiration, and her book is too. She cleverly blends together scientific evidence, practical exercises and amazing real life stories. I like books that make me stop and think, and this book certainly did that. This is a book that is about a way of being, a way to live our life from the heart, and shows how incredible that is. I would highly recommend it - it is a resource that you can keep and dip into for inspiration and as a reminder of how to live your life with heart.

Angela McCusker, mindfulness leader, teacher and speaker

This is an enlightening and heartfelt book that's hard to put down. Alisoun beautifully weaves insights, science and inspirational stories together in a way that prompts you to think differently about the part you play in creating your own happiness and success.

Julie Begbie, owner of Theta Jewellery and trainer

This book is a wellspring of ancient wisdom back by modern day science that shows how every one of us can live with Heartatude. An easy, inspiring and insightful read packed with helpful guidance and practical resources.

Fiona Ogg, founder of Lead A Bright Future

Heartatude is one of these books you just do not want to put down. Alisoun has such an easy to read approach that made her messages clear and understandable - I loved it! This book is a gift of knowledge I will refer to though out my life and I will share with others. The icing on the cake is that your journey doesn't stop when you finish this book, it's only just starting.

Heather McLennan, artist

Heartatude is an excellent read that unveils what we have always known in our hearts. It's full of practical advice on how to change your life by taking responsibility for your thoughts and emotions. Heartatude demands to be practiced and read continually.

Lucy MacLennan, lightworker

Contents

Foreword by Dr Lori Leyden PhD — **17**

Foreword by Dr David Hamilton PhD — **20**

Introduction — **23**

Part 1 – Heartatude

Chapter 1 – Why? — **33**

What is Success?
The 6 Factors That Determine Your Success
How Embracing Heartatude Will Help You

Chapter 2 – What is Heartatude? — **43**

The Heart-Centered Success Formula
The 9 Principles of Heart-Centered Success

Chapter 3 – An Evolving Science — **51**

From Whacky to Curiosity
Your Heart is More Than Just a Pump
The Powerhouse of Your Brain
The Relationship Between Your Heart and Your Brain
The Emergence of Heart Intelligence
The Mind/Body Connection
What You Feel Matters
Your Environment Often Matters More Than Your Genes
Even the 'Laws' of Physics Change
What Comes First – Science or Reality?

Part 2 – The 9 Principles Of Heart-Centered Success

Chapter 4 – Principle 1 – Engage Your Heart — **65**

Chapter 5 – Heart Value – Love — **70**

Ways to Enjoy More Love
Simple Ways to Demonstrate Love

Resourceful Questions, Affirmations, Tapping Statements &
Resources

Chapter 6 – Heart Value – Kindness   79

Ways to Be More Kind (to yourself and others)
Resourceful Questions, Affirmations, Tapping Statements &
Resources

Chapter 7 – Heart Value – Compassion   86

Ways to Be Compassionate (to yourself and others)
Resourceful Questions, Affirmations, Tapping Statements &
Resources

Chapter 8 – Heart Value – Integrity   93

How to Be More Aligned to Your Truth
Resourceful Questions, Affirmations, Tapping Statements &
Resources

Chapter 9 – Heart Value – Respect   98

How to Respect Yourself and Being Assertive
Tips for Respecting Others With Heart
Resourceful Questions, Affirmations, Tapping Statements &
Resources

Chapter 10 – Heart Value – Gratitude   106

Ways to Feel Grateful
Ways to Express Gratitude
Resourceful Questions, Affirmations, Tapping Statements &
Resources

Chapter 11 – Heart Value – Peace   113

How to Enjoy More Peace in Your Life
Resourceful Questions, Affirmations, Tapping Statements &
Resources

Chapter 12 – Principle 2 – Make a Difference   119

The Giving Spectrum
Knowing Your 'Why' – the Big Picture
Small Changes can Make a Huge Difference
Making a Difference to Yourself

Making a Difference to Others
Resourceful Questions, Affirmations, Tapping Statements & Resources

Chapter 13 – Principle 3 – Be the Masterful Authentic Leader You Were Born to Be   129

Identify What Makes You Unique
Get Clear on Your Purpose
Create a Compelling Vision
Define an Exciting Goal
Plan to Make it Happen
Overcome Any Beliefs or Feelings Limiting Your Success
Take Inspired Action
Resourceful Questions, Affirmations, Tapping Statements & Resources

Chapter 14 – Principle 4 – Embrace Personal Leadership & Responsibility   141

It's Your Choice
Your Genes Don't Always Control Your Health
You are Shaping Your Reality
Playing the Lead Role in Your Life
Resourceful Questions, Affirmations, Tapping Statements & Resources

Chapter 15 – Principle 5 – Manage Your Emotions   151

What You Feel Matters When it Comes to Success
Managing How You Feel in The Moment
Overcoming Negative Emotions
Creating Lasting Change
Resourceful Questions, Affirmations, Tapping Statements & Resources

Chapter 16 – Principle 6 – Invite Possibility & Success   169

What's Possible?
Developing a Success Mind-set
Embarking upon Your 'Hero's Journey'
How to Enjoy More Possibility & Success

Resourceful Questions, Affirmations, Tapping Statements & Resources

Chapter 17 – Principle 7 – Act Consciously with Positive Intention 179

Turning Off Your Auto-Pilot
The Scope of Intention
The 5 Steps to Taking Conscious Action
It's OK to Get it Wrong Sometimes
Defusing Others' Negative Behaviours With Intention
Resourceful Questions, Affirmations, Tapping Statements & Resources

Chapter 18 – Principle 8 – Develop Meaningful Connections & Relationships 188

The State of Healthy Relationships
Your Relationship With Yourself
Choosing Harmonious Relationships With Others
Your Relationship With Other Aspects of Life (Money, Success, Nature and the Planet)
Resourceful Questions, Affirmations, Tapping Statements & Resources

Chapter 19 – Principle 9 – Nurture & Tap into Natural Energy Resources for Peak Performance 201

Fuelling Your Body for Success
Other Natural Energy Sources
Managing Your Energy Vibration
Trusting Your Instincts
Creating Coincidences
The Law of Attraction
Unlimited Resources and Potential
How to Raise Your Energy Vibration
Resourceful Questions, Affirmations, Tapping Statements & Resources

Part 3 – Change Your Future

Chapter 20 – Take Enlightened Action 221

Developing Your Own Success Formula
The 7 Steps to Happiness and Success
The Power of Practice
Your Mind/Body Detox
Manifesting Miracles
Your Future is in Your Hands

A Few Closing Thoughts… 228

Part 4 – Resource Kit

Chapter 21 – Affirmations 233

How to Re-programme Your Mind
Using Affirmations
How to Create Your Own Affirmations
Ways to Get Results From Affirmations
How Long Does it Take for Affirmations to Work?

Chapter 22 – Tapping 239

What is Tapping?
How Does it Work?
How to Tap
Using Tapping for Success

Recommended Resources 245

Books, Films & Reports
List of Practical Heartatude Tools
Alisoun's Website
Other Resources

About the Author 247

Dedication

This book is dedicated to my gran, Elaine Wilson, who inspired me in so many ways to become the person I am today.

Appreciation

There are so many people who have contributed to me writing this book that I'd love to thank – so if you've been part of my journey in any way, I'm sending lots of hugs your way!

Particularly to those who have supported me over the last few years – my gorgeous husband Paul (I bet you're glad the writing of this is over); my mum, dad, family and friends, who have always been there; to all the kindred spirits who had faith in me and who have been instrumental in me reinventing a happier and more authentic life and career since 2003, including Fiona Ogg, Graeme Skea, Mary McPherson, David Hamilton, Lori Leyden, Bonnie Clarke and Dawn Breslin; all my clients; the Project LIGHT Rwanda Team and ambassadors; and of course, special thanks, too, to everyone who has helped turn this book into reality – my editor Christine McPherson, Kim and Sinclair Macleod from Indie Authors World, Deanna Evertt who designed the beautiful front cover and graphics, and to all my friends who gave lots of constructive feedback on the first few drafts.

With lots of love

Alisoun x

Foreword by Dr Lori Leyden PhD

In times of great intensity and chaos we have two choices – to see the nightmare of life unfolding or to focus on becoming part of the dream of what life can be. Out of chaos great change and innovation can arise. That's why I believe the stakes for attaining success are changing dramatically. When we become disillusioned or despairing and we fear that our hearts may be about to break, that can be the very time that our egos fall away and our hearts break open to new ways of being and doing in our personal and business lives.

In June 2010, I experienced a professional and personal betrayal that, while it did not break my heart, it did put me in a place I call a crisis of imagination. I had created a non-profit organisation called Create Global Healing to support my trauma healing work in Rwanda with orphan genocide survivors. Fundraising was always a difficult task for me because I just wanted to put all that energy into my work. I was very excited that the previous three years of networking, establishing the credibility of our work, and visioning my dream of Project LIGHT: Rwanda – the world's first international youth healing, leadership and entrepreneurship program – had great potential for being funded.

Long story short, I realized that a beloved friend whom I had introduced to many of my contacts was in fact using them to fund and support her own projects and hiding this from me. The details don't matter, but the deep disappointment, anger and fear that I felt was blocking me from imagining how I could ever create a new path for keeping my vision alive.

Well, as I had learned and committed myself to doing, I knew that forgiveness was necessary – forgiving this person, the situation, and most importantly myself. As I sat in deep meditation and moved through my forgiveness work, I imagined I was standing at the edge of my imagination for what was next on my path. Then I opened my heart to as much gratitude, love, joy and wonder as I could summon from the great release of forgiveness I had just experienced, and simply enjoyed how good it felt to return to a state I call grace.

Without effort, these quiet knowing words came to me – you just need to send out your heart-inspired vision into the Universe and all the right hearts will align with you... Really? How was that going to help me? Then I began to notice a celestial image forming in my heart-mind's eye – a rather ethereal 'movie' began to play out, and hearts began lighting up in the sky as the movie played on.

For the next several weeks I simply focused on my own heart connecting to and lighting up all the right hearts. In that time we completed a fundraising video that I sent out to people in the EFT/Tapping world and, while it would take me a while to make the connection, an Internet newsletter with a list of several hundred thousand subscribers featured the video that summer. The newsletter is put out by EFT Universe – no kidding!

Shortly thereafter, I received an email from a woman in Scotland named Alisoun Mackenzie. We Skyped in August and in October she miraculously joined our team in Rwanda. Months later, I met my new benefactor, Nick Ortner of the Tapping Solution, and by May 2011 Project LIGHT: Rwanda was a reality.

What does my story have to do with inspiring you to read this book?

First, when I look for a teacher or a partner in life or business, I look for a person who has the courage to be a spiritual adventurer and a pioneer of the hidden power of the heart to manifest personal and financial success. I encourage you to do the same. If you're reading these words, you've already found such a teacher.

Before you can write an exceptional, authentic book about heart-centered success, you first have to experience the path and embody the principles of getting there. Alisoun Mackenzie is 'Heartatude' in action. If you commit to the 9 Principles offered in this book, you will have an experiential roadmap to becoming a pioneer in co-creating a new paradigm for heart-centered success.

Join us in this new paradigm for healing ourselves, our children and our world.

Dr Lori Leyden, PhD, MBA

Trauma healing professional, author & speaker. Founder of *Create Global Healing* and partner of *The Tapping Solution Foundation.*

www.lorileyden.com

www.CreateGlobalHealing.org

www.ProjectLIGHTRwanda.com

www.TappingSolutionFoundation.org

Foreword by Dr David Hamilton PhD

Your thoughts and feelings shape your world. They determine what you do and your experience of life.

But they don't just influence your reality – they also impact the lives of others, too. Science shows that your thoughts and feelings are contagious. So whether you're happy or sad, loving or angry, what you're feeling rubs off on others.

It's a bit like being a radio transmitter interacting with people and the Universe around you. What you send and receive depends upon your signal. If you're embroiled in negativity, judgment or fear, this will be reflected in your day-to-day reality. However, when you act from a place of love, kindness and compassion, you'll have a very different experience. What type of beacon do you want to be – one who finds it easier or harder to attract success?

I'm always inspired and moved by the stories Alisoun shares about her experiences helping genocide survivors in Rwanda. The transformations of those who have been through some of the worst horrors imaginable are remarkable, and exemplify the power of love, compassion, gratitude and belief. That miracles happen when we connect to our soul, have faith in ourselves, open our hearts to love and take inspired action.

Alisoun calls this alignment Heartatude, and in this thought-provoking book she shares how you too can reconnect to the true essence of who you are, enjoy more happiness, and meaningful success.

Be ready to enjoy a journey through The 9 Principles Of Heart-Centered Success that will touch your heart and open your mind to new possibilities. This isn't a book that prescribes all the answers. Rather, Alisoun masterfully offers ideas and questions for you to think about in the context of making authentic changes in your life or overcoming problems you face. This is a wonderful practical guide that challenges you to consider what success really means to you and how best to achieve this.

Your future is in your hands – enjoy!

Dr David Hamilton PhD Scientist, author & speaker

www.drdavidhamilton.com

It's The Thought That Counts, How Your Mind Can Heal Your Body, Why Kindness Is Good For You, & more

Introduction

'Excellence is not an act, it is a habit.'
Aristotle

What one thing in your life would you love to change?

Every single moment is a unique opportunity for you to make a choice that will profoundly change the rest of your life. You make choices that impact your future all the time – but do they take you nearer to your destiny or soul purpose?

One of the most inspiring people I've ever met is a young man called Matteui, who was only eight at the time of the Rwandan genocide in 1994. His mum had died, and so he was brought up by his grieving father and elder brother.

Living on a remote mountain farm, it took a great deal of effort just to survive – working long hours on the land and often only having one meal of rice a day. Their small house had no running water, electricity, or any of the comforts most in developed countries enjoy.

From a young age Matteui dreamt of a better life for him and his family, and decided the way to do this was to get a good education. He would get up at 5am to walk for two hours to and from school each day, wearing only flip-flops on his feet. His family didn't have the money to pay for food during the day, so often he would go hungry. Sometimes he wasn't allowed to attend classes because he didn't have any money to pay the fees, so he stood outside listening. Yet he persevered and remarkably completed high school.

But then, as a young adult in a country with few jobs, Matteui began to doubt whether he'd ever be able to get a job or afford to go to university. Until he joined Project LIGHT Rwanda – a programme I'm involved in where we show young genocide survivors how to overcome their trauma and become heart-centered leaders in their community. Having completed the programme, Matteui is now at university and feels he's living his dream.

His sheer grit, determination, and commitment are inspiring. But what's even more humbling is the pure love and gratitude that oozes from every cell in his body, which he summed up beautifully recently when he said, 'Life is better when you are happy but life is the best when other people are happy because of you. Give peace and share your smile with everyone.'

Just imagine what you could achieve if you applied the same love and determination to all you do…

I remember a few years ago feeling something was missing in my life. To those looking in from the outside, my life looked great – it appeared I was happily married, enjoying a good social life, had a successful career and I was fit and healthy. But I felt empty inside. And I didn't know why, let alone what to do about it.

I didn't feel like I was making a valuable contribution to society through my work, and spending money on things I didn't need to bring fleeting moments of happiness seemed like madness. I yearned for something better – a way of life where I could be happy each day, not just at the weekend or when I was on holiday. One where I felt connected to a sense of purpose and to be making a real difference in the world rather than having to compromise what was important to me.

But is that possible?

What would people think?

How could I make that happen?

By contrast, I was recently overwhelmed by a deep sense of happiness I felt inside as I walked along a beach near my home – I was basked in gratitude as I realised I felt my body was full of contentment and happiness despite the chaos of what was happening that day. There were things I would have loved to be different, but I didn't 'need' anything else to be happy. Something had changed within me, but what?

As is often the case, something unexpected is the catalyst for change, e.g. the feelings that erupt upon the birth of a child, illness or injury, the death of a loved one, an unexpected windfall, the breakdown of a relationship, burnout, children leaving home, the loss of a job, insolvency of a business, or retirement.

For me it was the opportunity of redundancy (or severance, as I think it is called in the US). I had two options – to continue my dull existence in an alien environment that fuelled an unsustainable lifestyle; or to invite the curious part of me to be brave and come out to play. I began to wonder whether I could create a lifestyle that would bring me a deeper sense of happiness, self-worth, and meaningful success. I could feel a glimmer of hope inside and knew redundancy was too good an opportunity to miss. And so in 2003, I stepped into the world of personal development and self-employment.

If you knew it was possible to change one thing in your life, would you do it?

The purpose of this book is to give you ideas how you can put yourself in the best place to succeed in whatever way is important to you – whether this is in your personal life, your work, or your business. And to effectively overcome any challenges you encounter. I don't claim to know all the answers, but instead present this collection of insights, information, resources and questions with a view to stimulating your ideas on how best to approach your success and cope with life's challenges.

By embracing what I share, you'll find it easier to naturally attract more happiness and success with less effort. You're also likely to find that your energy, physical, and emotional wellbeing will improve too.

Throughout this book you'll not only learn many practical tools you can use to boost how you feel and the results you get, you'll also learn the science supporting many of them. And how adopting a heart-centered approach to life also enhances the lives of those around you.

I've been greatly influenced by the young genocide survivors I've worked with in Rwanda, who have taught me so much about the capacity we all have within us to pick ourselves up and embrace life, no matter what we've experienced. The model of Heartatude I present in this book brings together much of what is taught in the Western world plus what I've learnt from different cultures around the world.

When you align your life to the core essence of who you are and act from a place of love, joy and peace in your heart, you will attract more of what you want. By contrast, when you are disconnected from your natural spirit, or act from a place of fear, lack, resentment or frustration, you often unintentionally attract more of what you say you don't want at a conscious level.

When you adopt a heart-centered approach, life's challenges still happen but you may experience fewer of these and be better able to cope with them when you do.

How to Get The Most from This Book

Collectively, the content of this book is a compilation of the best tools I've learnt for creating a joyful and rewarding life, and for coping better with any curve balls that life throws at you. The simple strategies I share have already transformed the lives of many of my clients.

The book is split into four parts:

Part 1 – Heartatude

Discover the key components of this approach to success, how it works, and the supporting science.

Part 2 – The 9 Principles of Heart-Centered Success

Learn these simple principles and supporting practical tools you can use to immediately boost your happiness and success. The techniques I share are a selection of the personal development tools and spiritual practices which have helped me to grow personally over the last few years, and which have also been transformational for my clients.

Because different things work for each of us, I encourage you to try them out and then develop new habits for using the ones that work best for you.

The practical exercises are a mix of those that relate directly to each principle, plus examples of powerful interventions you can use to be more effective in any situation. The latter includes:

- **Resourceful Questions**

   The brain is a phenomenal storehouse of all your personal experiences and also a very obedient servant, once you know how to 'work it' effectively. All you need to do is to learn how to tap into the power of your mind and the mind/body connection, to boost your success. One of the easiest ways to do this is to direct your mind to focus on a particular task, or to come up with an answer to a specific question.

   You'll therefore find 'resourceful questions' to ask yourself at the end of each chapter in Part 2, to raise your awareness about the part you are playing in creating your experience or life. And to help you come up with great ideas to help you meet your desired outcomes in any situation.

- **Empowering Affirmations**

An affirmation is simply a statement; although, in this context I mean positive statements you can say to yourself repeatedly to re-programme your mind for success.

I explain more about how to define and maximise your success with affirmations in Chapter 21, and I've listed suggested affirmations at the end of each chapter for you to use or adapt.

- **Transformational 'Tapping' Statements**

One of the most incredible techniques I've discovered that anyone can easily learn to change how they think and feel (physically, emotionally and energetically), is 'tapping' (e.g. Emotional Freedom Technique (EFT)). It's also very effective for pain and trauma relief, and is the main technique that has helped the genocide survivors we work with in Rwanda, to let go of the past and to embrace new and brighter futures.

I explain 'tapping' in more detail in Chapter 22 and list transformational tapping statements at the end of each chapter, to assist you in using this technique.

Part 3 – Choose Your Future

Get ideas on how to apply these principles to help you feel good, achieve your goals, and manifest miracles.

Part 4 – Resource Kit

Find out more about more about tapping, affirmations, and other resources to help you on your journey.

Thereafter, I invite you to dip into the relevant chapters of this book whenever you are faced with a challenge, want to create a change, or work towards a goal – to treat this book as a nourishing success toolkit.

Your On-line Questionnaire

In Chapter 2, I refer you to a questionnaire that you can download from my website, to find out which of the 9 Principles it would be beneficial for you to concentrate on first; those which, once mastered, could have the greatest potential positive outcomes.

I invite you to use this questionnaire as a guide to track your personal development progress. You could print it off and do it today, and again regularly (e.g. each month), so that you have more awareness of what's influencing how you are feeling, the progress you're making, and how you are taking control of the results you're getting. Just like doing a regular health check.

Website (www.alisoun.com/heartatude)

At the end of some chapters, I refer you to further tools, resources, and information that you can find on my website. I invite you to go to the relevant links to connect, listen to the audios, download the practical exercises, or sign up to receive regular updates from me.

Your Personal Success Journal

Journaling is a great way to clear your mind, stimulate new ideas, and recognise how the action you're taking is having an impact on the results you're getting.

And so I encourage you to get a special notebook that you can use to note down your thoughts and key nuggets as you read through this book.

I'll be sharing lots of ideas for the type of things you may wish to reflect on and note in this journal, including the practical exercises I share.

True Stories

Throughout this book I'll be sharing many true stories about those who are ambassadors for adopting a 'Heartatude' approach to life; my own personal life experiences, and of people I have met and who have inspired me. The purpose of sharing these with you is to demonstrate how the principles and tools I teach can be applied for maximum impact. In several cases I have changed the names to respect confidentiality.

How Long Does it Take to Be Successful?

People sometimes ask me how long it will take to achieve their goals, or to implement the changes they'd like to make. That's a bit like asking someone how long it will take to clear your garden of weeds when they haven't seen the size and state of the garden!

So while the tools and techniques I share are easy to learn and will help you be happier and succeed more quickly (than continuing to do what hasn't been working), the results you get will depend on the effort you put into changing yourself.

Whatever you're looking to change, your current situation is – to some extent – a reflection of how you have thought, felt, and acted until today.

Do you ever look back at a hairdo or outfit which used to make you feel and look fantastic, and cringe? If you can change your mind about something that used to make you feel great, you can change what's not working for you too.

If you simply read the book but don't make any alterations to the way you approach life, you're unlikely to notice any significant changes. To get the best results, you need to actually change something about what you're doing. And, where relevant, to replace habits that are sabotaging your happiness or success with those that will propel you forward.

So the time it takes to achieve your goals, feel better or cope better depends on your starting point relative to what you want – and the commitment you've got to make it happen. You'll be able to change some things quickly, but you may have some stubborn weeds that will take a little more effort to pull out.

Those who benefit most from what I share are those who commit to investing in themselves – by setting aside the time to read the whole of this book, by practising the techniques that resonate most with them, and by following up the resources I share that are of most interest to them.

The type of interventions you choose for your journey also influence how long it takes – are you going to walk, drive, or go by plane? When you use resources that work at a subconscious level (e.g. tapping, NLP or hypnosis), learn more skills, and are savvy in the strategies you adopt, you will speed up your journey.

I hope you enjoy the book, and wish you every success in the future.

Alisoun x

January 2015

Your Invitation To Connect

I'd love to hear your thoughts as you read through this book, and of any success stories that you have from applying any of what I share.

Check out www.alisoun.com/heartatude for details of how to connect with me.

PART 1

- Heartatude -

Chapter 1

Why?

'May it be said, when the sun sets on your life, you made a difference.'
Mac Anderson, Business Leader & Author

Imagine feeling a deep sense of peace and being able to create the life you'd love for yourself and others in a way that reflects the true essence of who you are – that natural spirit you were born to be. A life where:

• you enjoy an abundant flow of love, happiness and success.

• you are loved for just being you.

• you are appreciated for your efforts.

• you feel energised and invigorated about life.

• you are making a difference in a way that matters.

• you are in a good state of physical and emotional health.

• your actions enrich the lives of others, just as the sun brings life to the planet.

Of course, you are already a special blessing to the world, no matter how you feel about what's happening in your life right now. You are love. Love exists within you. It's always there, even in times when you can't feel it. You deserve to be happy. To be loved. And to be successful – in whatever way is important to you.

We live in such exciting times of change and endless possibilities – if you choose to push through your comfort zone and neutralise any fears or anxieties by reconnecting with the natural abundant flow of love within your heart. And to re-align all you are and all you do around this.

In 2010, I decided to go Rwanda to be involved in a humanitarian project with genocide survivors. We teach these incredible young people trauma healing, heart-centered leadership, and entrepreneurial skills.

These exceptionally kind and loving people have taught me so much about human beings' resilience and our capacity to survive. My experiences with them over the last few years have enhanced my life in so many ways, and reminded me of what's genuinely important.

To have witnessed, as young children, the murder of their families and to have then brought themselves up – many with little adult intervention, money or food – is beyond miraculous. Their ability to survive despite the trauma and hardship they experienced, to forgive one another, to work collaboratively, and to live in peace, is truly remarkable.

Undoubtedly, many of the Rwandan people who were around during and just after the 1994 genocide are still highly traumatised. But most of those we've been working with no longer experience the same emotional distress.

Their ability to feel forgiveness in their hearts towards those who committed such horrific murderous acts, demonstrates that we all have the capacity to forgive; to move forward with love and peace in our hearts. And if these young people can release their trauma, anger and despair, then we, too, have the potential to heal our own emotional scars and triggers.

Around the capital, Kigali, you often hear the wonderful uplifting melodies of people singing in churches and see adults congregating in the streets, while children run around happily playing with whatever they can lay their hands on.

There is a thirst to significantly improve their living conditions, education and jobs, and to become a thriving economy. Yet many live without the basics most of us in developed countries are accustomed to, such as running water, electricity, a variety of food choices, entertainment or furniture.

When I ask how they cope with what they've experienced, comments include, 'God has spared me, I am alive' or 'My hope is to spread more love and light in the world, so genocide never happens again'.

Many appear happier, more loving, expressive of gratitude, community-focussed, proactive and more optimistic than large pockets of Western societies, who seem to moan and complain about trivia with little sense of personal responsibility.

Their affectionate expressions of love, curiosity for life, willingness to learn and adapt to an ever-changing environment, continues to inspire me. And I'm so grateful to them for opening my mind to the potential that's within us all.

What is Success?

One of the ways the Collins' Dictionary describes success is 'the attainment of wealth or fame'. But there is no mention of love, happiness or peace. Yet when we strive for success, it's often the benefits of achieving our goals that we're really aspiring to enjoy, e.g. the happiness, confidence or sense of self-worth.

I wonder what would be different if our children were taught from an early age to aspire to be happy, loving or kind – not just through formal teaching, but in the way they experience emotions, well-being, behaviours, and the actions of all those around them.

What would our society be like if wealth, status and possessions were by-products of being happy, rather than perceived routes to happiness (that often don't deliver)?

In his book, *Success Intelligence*, Robert Holden talks about 'insanity of success' – the way that so many people pursue success as a primary goal, sacrificing health, marriages, and many other positive life experiences, in the pursuit of something many don't ever feel they achieve.[1]

In 1972, King Jigme Singye Wangchuck of Bhutan declared Gross National Happiness (helping those within a nation to be happy) to be more important than Gross National Product (simply measuring what a population produces). And from that time, Bhutan oriented their national policy and development around this.[2]

A definition I like is one presented by Dr David Hawkins in his book *Power Vs. Force* – 'true success enlivens and supports the spirit; it has nothing to do with isolated achievements, but instead relates to being accomplished as a total person, and attaining a lifestyle that benefits not only the individual, but everyone around them.'[3]

---

1 *Success Intelligence*, Robert Holden, Hay House, 2008, pxiii

2 *A Short Guide To Gross National Happiness*, URA, ALRKIRE, ZANGMO & WANGDI, The Centre For Bhutan Studies, 2012, p6

3 *Power Vs Force*, Dr David R. Hawkins, Hay House, 2002, p203.

Or, as one of my business mentors George Kao says, 'true success is spiritual growth through the path of altruistic or selfless service.'

Personally, I believe success is the ability to feel love and contentment in your heart, be a true expression of yourself, and have a positive impact in the world.

For the purposes of this book, feel free to define success in whatever way is important to you. This could relate to your family, attaining goals, sporting achievements, your dream job, being in a wonderful relationship, living in your own home, having a good social life, something health-related, doing voluntary work, or some form of spiritual connection.

It's OK to set yourself financial goals to meet, e.g. to pay for a holiday, or save up for a deposit for a property, or other material goods. Sometimes it is the 'responsible' thing to do. But remember that success is far more than just being about money, status or fame – particularly for the larger goals in life. Sometimes it's also worth exploring whether there are other ways to experience the desired outcomes you think the attainment of money, promotion, or fame will bring, e.g. happiness, freedom, choice, or security.

What does success mean to you?

• How do you want to feel?

• What type of person do you want to be?

• What impact do you want to make?

• Do you want to succeed the easy or the hard way?

• What would you like others to be saying about you today?

• What would you like others to be saying about you at your funeral?

• What would you like to achieve?

• What kind of people do you like being around?

When I ask the last question at workshops I've run, the personal qualities that often come up are people who are honest, trustworthy, fun, kind, caring, have similar values, opinions, and ethics. And those who are positive and proactive.

If any of these appeal to you, adopting a heart-centred approach to success is likely to be one of the most authentic and fulfilling ways for you to feel good, exhibit these qualities, and succeed.

The 6 Factors That Determine Your Success

The following six factors underpin The 9 Principles of Heart-Centered Success, and form the basis for the tools and techniques that you'll learn throughout this book:

1. Your thoughts and feelings

You'll know from your own experience that the way you feel has a huge impact on how you interact with others and what you do.

Has there ever been a time when you've consciously wanted to say something but your feelings, such as nerves, doubts or anxieties, have held you back from speaking up? Or you've known what to do, but haven't done it?

What you think influences how you feel. What you feel drives your actions. Your actions (what you do and how you act) influence how others perceive you, and ultimately the results you get.

It's therefore critical for you to develop a mind-set and emotional capacity for success, and all that you associate with it.

2. Your actions

Do you ever come up with an idea or set yourself a goal to achieve, but then take action that is not aligned to this? And if so, is it any surprise that you don't then end up with the success you desire?

Those who succeed generally take a proactive, positive, and focussed approach to success. They take the time to define the outcomes they want; planning how they will achieve these, e.g. getting all the resources they need in place such as time, money, materials and support; and then taking action aligned to what they've decided to work towards. However, others may set out with positive intentions or goals but then give in to subconscious habits and behaviours which sabotage their success.

Consciously switching off your autopilot and doing something aligned to what you'd like to achieve, is one of the principles I'll come on to later.

3. Your personal brand

What I mean by this is what other people think, feel, and say about you – inwardly, to your face, or when you are out of the room.

This is important, because others' perceptions of you will have a huge impact on your day-to-day experiences and the results you get.

People are happier to spend time with, help out, work with, work for, and buy from, people who they know, like and trust. This 'liking' and 'trusting' comes from their perception of who you are, such as: what you do; what you don't do; the way you express yourself; how you treat others; what they see you prioritising; the consistency of what you say versus what you do; and the quality of your outputs.

You are effectively a walking, talking brand.

Every single time you are visible to others (and particularly to those you'd like to influence), it's critical that you make sure the 'messages' you project (through your words, tonality, body language, actions, and behaviours) are congruent with:

- who you are and the 'brand' you'd like to put out there

- what you want others to be saying about you

- what you want others to be feeling when they are around you

- what they feel when they experience your friendship, love, attention, support, help, products, or services.

The good news is that by mastering The 9 Principles of Heart-Centered Success, you'll be far more likely to get this right. You will then increase the likelihood that you'll be perceived as a kind, compassionate, confident, trustworthy, reliable and smart person who people will want to connect with, help, be around, work alongside, buy from, and have fun with. This will, in turn, mean you are far more likely to attract more success with less effort on a day-to-day basis.

4. Your personal energy

Has there ever been a time when you've met somebody who has said all the right things but there was something about them that you didn't resonate with? You may not have known why exactly, but you just knew there was something about them you didn't like or trust.

You'll hopefully also have had many other experiences of connecting easily with people you have met. People you feel good to be around; ideas and chat flow easily between you; you feel energised; you feel naturally inclined to spend time with them and to support them; and you know the connection is mutual.

In both cases, what you've experienced has been personal energy – your energy and the energy of others. This always influences how you feel and respond to others. And likewise, how others react to you.

From a scientific perspective, you, me, everything around us is simply a mass of vibrating molecules. We are all what may appear to the human eye as separate beings, but at subatomic level we are simply part of a greater mass of energy. We are all clusters of energy that collectively form one universe.

Every single thought you have has energy associated with it, as does every emotion you feel. Since we are all part of a greater oneness, what you think and feel will therefore not only have an impact on you but also on other people, on other living creatures, objects, and things around you.

Whether or not you are consciously 'managing' your personal energy, you are sending off energy vibes to those around you. And your personal energy has a direct result on much of what you attract in life.

So if you want to attract more happiness and success in your life, it's about raising your energy vibration to do this. Mastering the 9 Principles I share in this book will enable you do this.

5. Your contribution

While having personal goals will boost the likelihood of your success, to some extent you also have a dependency upon others and a responsibility towards this amazing planet we inhabit.

It is within your nature as a human being to be loving, caring and kind. And when you are connected to your natural way of being, your actions will also have a positive impact on your family, friends, community and world. However, sometimes we can allow our ego to distract us from what's really important in life and cause us not to notice what's going on around us, e.g. when you're attached to checking out what's happening on your mobile phone, you're missing out on all sorts of possibilities for connecting with others and being human.

Is how you spend your time having a positive or negative impact on those around you and who are important to you?

Your happiness and success is closely linked to the contribution you make towards your own happiness and success plus that of others.

6. Your connection

Your level of connection to the pure essence of who you are, to nature, and to the infinite possibilities of the greater universe, all have an impact on the type of success you experience. The more connected you are, the more satisfying, rewarding, and peaceful your journey of life in this physical realm will be.

Whether or not you are fully aware of the consequences of being you – your thoughts do matter. Your feelings matter. Your actions matter. Because you are part of the Universe, you are always influencing others, animals and the ecosystem of the world. We are all part of one universe. We are not separate.

Collectively, the energy of the 7+ billion people who inhabit this planet today is influencing our day-to-day experience of life and the legacy we are leaving for our children. I share more on this throughout this book.

How Embracing 'Heartatude' Will Help You

The 9 Principles of Heart-Centered Success that form the basis of Heartatude give you the knowledge and tools to put you in the best place to succeed, irrespective of your dreams, background, life so far or starting point today. If you embrace them, you will:

• find it easier to get the results that you want and attract more success

• feel happier and healthier on a day-to-day basis

• feel more aligned with the true essence of who you are

• connect and relate well with others in a way that matters

• be able to let go of doubts, worries, anxieties, and fears that hold you back from getting the results you want

• respond more calmly, confidently, and effectively to challenging people and situations

• have more of a positive impact on others

• be a more influential player

• enjoy harmonious relationships

- have greater peace of mind

- avoid making costly and time-consuming mistakes

- be happier at work in a way that doesn't compromise what's important to you

- be able to earn good money doing what you love

- have more time, energy, and money to spend with family, friends, and doing what's important to you.

And when things get tough, you'll also be able to overcome these challenges more easily.

Personally, I've used the approach and tools I share with you in this book to navigate my way through several testing times over the last ten years – to turn redundancy into one of the best things that happened to me; to overcome the disappointment of not having children; to come through a divorce with only love in my heart for my ex-husband; and to learn to sleep at night again, having built up a property portfolio (with debt) just before the property crash in 2008.

While going through each of these events, I noticed that while they challenged me emotionally, the tools I used enabled me to cope better than many people in similar positions. I hate to think of people feeling stuck, miserable, or overwhelmed with what they are facing, which is why I've decided to share with you the best of what I've learned.

For centuries many people have focussed on working towards 'having' rather than 'being'; on 'winning' at a cost to others; 'taking' rather than 'giving'; or 'giving' too much to others, at a personal cost to themselves.

The 9 Principles are an invitation for equilibrium, based on some of the latest scientific knowledge, ancient wisdom, spiritual practices and current transformational tools. By mastering these Principles, you'll enjoy a healthy balance between getting your own needs met and making a difference to others. You'll also open the door to abundance – not just in terms of wealth, but in all aspects of life.

Thankfully, there is a growing swell of people who not only want to succeed for personal gain but who also want to transform the lives of others and make the world a better place. A shift in attitudes and consciousness has already started, with communities around the world being energised by this ethos and potential.

One of my favourite quotes is from someone who continually pushes the realms of possibility and success, and is also a leading visionary and philanthropist – Richard Branson. In his book 'Screw Business As Usual', the philosophy he shares is 'do good, have fun, and the money will come'.4 This is certainly the approach I aim to adopt in all that I do in business, and I encourage you to do the same in the work you do, too.

---

4. *Screw Business As Usual, Richard Branson, 2011, Virgin Books, p8*

Your Invitation To Connect

If you like what you've read so far, I'd love to connect with you.

Check out www.alisoun.com/heartatude for details of how to connect with me and other like-minded people.

Chapter 2

What is Heartatude?

'Success comes from knowing that you did your best to become the best that you are capable of becoming.'
John Wooden, Basketball Coach

It was so heartening to hear what a friend's son of eight said, when asked what he wanted for Christmas. He simply replied, 'Peace in the world.' What makes this boy exceptional is that he not only said this but also took action aligned to his words. After taking the time to think about how he could make a difference, he went on to get the support of his head-teacher, other pupils, and parents, and held an African fair (selling baking and jewellery) at his school, in aid of the genocide survivors I work with in Rwanda. Shortly after, his classmates were asked to share who they admired and why. Many said their parents or gave the names of famous people. However, four classmates mentioned this young boy because, as they said, 'He is kind, and has the confidence to be himself.' I am filled with gratitude for all their efforts, and have faith that in the future people like this young boy will lead and inspire others to create a better world.

The Heart-Centered Success Formula

Heartatude offers an authentic, compassionate, and holistic approach to success. One that yields results through being true to yourself, engaging your heart, acting with integrity, striving for excellence, being of service to others, and making a positive contribution to the planet.

It is about aligning your head, heart and actions to your purpose, so that you channel your energy towards getting meaningful results and inspiring others to do the same. Collectively, these elements create your personal energy, which in turn influences, and is influenced by, the Universe of which we are all part.

Let me explain this in more detail:

- What I mean by 'purpose' is whatever gives your life meaning, e.g. your family, the contribution you make to society, your soul purpose or spiritual connection, a cause close to your heart, or what's important to you.

  Your purpose may be something that excites you, or you feel passionately about. Or it could be a mission you've embraced as a consequence of a challenging life experience, such as the illness or death of a loved one. You may have a purpose that is with you for life. Or you may engage with several in response to your life experiences.

  Your purpose is bigger than the roles and identities you take on in life, such as what you do, who you are in your family or community, what you have, and who you know.

  At a deeper level, your soul purpose is at the core of who you are. It is you in your purest form – your natural energy or life force that always exists. It is your natural spirit that has been part of you since before you were born, and continues in spirit once you leave this physical world. It's always part of you – even when you are unsure of who you are and when you doubt yourself. Some call this your soul, pure unconditional love, or your infinite or higher self. It's your inner guide that knows what's right for you. And through your body, it gives you feedback if all is not right in the form of intuition, negative feelings, and physical sensations or illness.

- When I say 'head' in the context of this model, I am referring to your thoughts (at both a conscious and unconscious level), and that includes your mind-set (beliefs), memories, knowledge, and skills. These could be the words, images, and movies you play in your mind, the associations you've created from your life experiences, and the software programmes you run in your mind that manifest as your actions and habits.

- Your 'heart' represents everything you love to do – the things that excite and energise you. It also signifies how you manage your feelings and tap into the natural power and intelligence of your heart.

- Actions are simply what you do (or don't do) and how you act.

To be as healthy, happy, resilient, and successful as you'd love to be, it's about aligning each of these four elements so they are working towards the same desired outcomes. And so you are omitting the energy that will help you attract more of what you'd like in the outer world, as well as to better cope with life's challenges.

However, many people say what they'd love to do or how they would love to be, but then spend their time and/or money taking action that is not aligned to this.

How many people do you know who are in jobs they hate because they don't know another way to earn their desired level of income? Or those who strive for life balance but do very little to look after themselves?

Have you ever set yourself a goal and then spent time doing something that ensures you don't achieve this? This could be to master a sport, to improve your health, to take up a new hobby, to set up a business, to get involved in a community project, to do something in your home, or to spend more special time with loved ones.

Often what you experience and the results you get are a good indication of whether each of these factors is in alignment or not, e.g. when you are working towards a goal, but have fear or anxiety in your heart, you are less likely to take the action required to achieve it. Do you have dreams you'd love to manifest, but allocate no time each day, week or month towards making these happen?

Because you are constantly interacting with and being influenced by the world around you, maintaining this alignment can be challenging. And sometimes when there is a huge gap between your head and your heart, the journey to alignment can seem like a long one. The starting point is to become more consciously aware of your thoughts, feelings, and actions, from today and on an on-going basis.

It was during a time of misalignment and overwhelm that I came up with what has since evolved into The 9 Principles of Heart-Centered Success.

I had built up a financially successful business but I was working extremely long hours and travelling too much. It wasn't the flexible and fun life I'd envisioned for myself when I started out.

When I stopped to consider the part I'd played in this, I recognised that I had become a slave to a job I'd created. I had succeeded in creating a reliable income by filling my training diary for the next six months. It felt good to have achieved one of my goals – to be able to support myself financially by doing something I loved – but I was knackered and felt trapped.

I'd allowed myself to be drawn into what other people thought I was good at and what they wanted me to do for them, rather than doing what nourished my soul and was going to be good for me – physically, emotionally and spiritually. As a consequence, I had become disconnected from the true essence of who I am, and from the more relaxed, fun, and financially abundant lifestyle I craved.

So I took the time to reconnect with my passions and to come up with a plan of how get back on track. To do this, I used the tools I'd found most effective during my years of personal development. And so the first seeds of Heartatude were sown.

You see, when your head, heart, and actions are not aligned to your purpose, you are likely to be manifesting things you don't want, such as unhappiness, challenging relationships, a lack of what you'd like, problems at work, and negative physical conditions.

I'm not talking about every bad experience that happens in your life, because there are many things that will shock, upset, or sadden you that you have no control over (or, at least, in the realms of this lifetime). And it's healthy to experience a full spectrum of emotions, including upset, grief or shock, in response to many of life's challenges. What I am referring to, however, are all the situations you do have control or influence over – those where you've played a part in creating the conditions you are faced with today. Even though it's hard to admit you've co-created at some level.

For example, when you are harbouring strong negative feelings such as fear, a lack of worthiness, anxiety, anger or resentment, if you don't acknowledge these feelings and take action to release these emotions, you are limiting your potential for happiness and success. And you could also be:

- living a life that doesn't completely reflect the true essence of who you are.

- wasting time doing things that keep your dreams at bay – at a cost to you and others.

- limiting the way you are able to support and help others.

- lowering your energy vibration, resulting in you attracting more of what you don't want in your life.

So how do you align each of these four components and attract more success?

The good news is that in the same way you've learned to be the person you are today, you can change whatever is not working so that you can create a different future for yourself and others.

On a recent trip to Rwanda, a new member of our team commented on the unusual energy of the young people we've been working with. She was particularly struck by the way that love, peace, and joy naturally radiate from every cell in their bodies, and the outward expressions of love and affection they display for one another. When we're with this group, spontaneous bursts of laughter, singing, dancing, clapping and prayer are the norm. They are both living proof and teachers of the capacity that we all have to heal ourselves and to attract miracles when we let go of the past, invite peace, and surrender to what has held us back.

Heartatude is underpinned by The 9 Principles of Heart-Centered Success that collectively provide a simple framework and practical tools for you to use. By mastering these 9 Principles, you will be able to recognise and correct any misalignment in your thoughts, feelings, and actions. You can then take remedial action and start to get better results.

These tools helped me to transform my life, have helped many of my clients, and also the young people in Rwanda.

The 9 Principles of Heart-Centered Success

Here is a brief summary of these principles that I cover in more detail in Part 2:

1. Engage Your Heart

In all you do – towards yourself, the way you connect with others and respond to situations:

- **Love – be the embodiment of love. Listen and be true to the inner guidance of your heart.**

- **Kindness – act with kindness and generosity.**

- **Compassion – connect with how all living creatures feel, and take action to eliminate suffering.**

- **Integrity – be true and authentic to the pure essence of who you were born to be.**

- **Respect – treat yourself with respect and be mindful of others' rights and opinions.**

- **Gratitude – be appreciative and express gratitude.**

- **Peace – release the past, be forgiving, and let go of future worries.**

2. Make a Difference

Align your actions to have a positive impact – for you, others, the world, and the planet. Stepping up to share your unique gifts, skills, and qualities in a way that you are of best support, service, or value to your family, clients, colleagues, organisation, or whatever cause is important to you.

3. Be The Masterful Authentic Leader You Were Born To Be

Proactively enhance your self-awareness and personal development to enable you to achieve results aligned to who you truly are, to have the greatest positive impact, and to inspire others to do the same.

4. Embrace Personal Leadership & Responsibility

Proactively direct your life by taking responsibility for choosing thoughts, feelings, and actions that will enable you to enjoy more meaningful success and inspire others to be the best they can be, too.

5. Manage Your Emotions

Manage your emotions effectively so you can choose to respond calmly to challenges and channel your energy towards the things you can control, so you create the best potential outcomes for you and those around you.

6. Invite Possibility & Success

Open your mind and be curious about the endless possibilities for your success. Choose empowering thoughts and take inspired action to create opportunities and manifest your goals.

7. Act Consciously with Positive Intention

Consciously choose the focus of your attention, define your desired outcomes and consider positive intentions ahead of responding to people/situations, and then consciously take action aligned to these.

8. Develop Meaningful Connections & Relationships

Reconnect with the inner essence of who you really are. Make time to relate and connect with others, to be truly present in their company, and to build harmonious and fruitful relationships with all you interact with.

9. Nurture and Tap into Natural Energy Resources for Peak Performance

Nurture, listen and respond to feedback from your heart, mind, body, soul, and universal intelligence for optimum performance, increased energy, longevity, and to attract what is in the highest good of you, others, and the planet.

These 9 Principles collectively represent a blueprint for your happiness, success, and ability to cope with life's challenges; how you embrace these influences; how you interact with the world; how you respond to life events and others; how others perceive you and feel around you; the impact you have; and the results you get.

One of my friends, Lorraine, is a wonderful heart-centered soul. Through being truly focused on expressing her authentic self and how she can help others, she has built a successful business, training people around the world and as an author. It's Lorraine's unique blend of a loving heart, hard work, business savvy, and the way she energetically walks her talk which have contributed to her success. I love the way her business has grown organically and evolved, by responding with love and peace to the needs of those around her and opportunities that have presented themselves. And, because she's a master of doing what it takes to raise her energy vibration, she seems to attract success with ease.

Whether you're looking to achieve a particular goal, to improve your happiness, health, life balance, to change direction, or looking for ideas on how to respond more effectively to challenges, these principles will guide you towards better choices. They enable you to work out what to focus on and the practical steps to take to achieve the best positive outcomes.

What I suggest you do is to apply these principles in relation to yourself, and then in an area of your life you'd like to change, or find challenging. By adopting a heart-centered approach to changing yourself, you will create a ripple effect of change for you and others, in ways that are important to you.

Download Your Heart-Centered Success Questionnaire

If you'd like to find out what it could be beneficial for you to focus on first to attract more success, you can download a simple questionnaire at **www.alisoun.com/heartatude**

Have fun!

Chapter 3

An Evolving Science

'The practice of science happens at the border between the known and the unknown. Standing on the shoulders of giants, we peer into the darkness with eyes opened not in fear but in wonder.'
Brian Cox, Scientist

Some of my fondest memories are those when I was a wee girl sitting on my gran's bed in Troon, watching her doing her hair. I adored my gran, and these were our special moments together – often just the two of us – before going downstairs to spend the rest of the day with the family. One of the regular topics of conversation was all the tiny bottles of white pills she kept in a cupboard. I was of an age where I'd been conditioned not to go through other people's things, or to take tablets unless adult members of my family gave them to me, and so I was curious about these. I didn't understand much about them, other than they were wonder pills she'd give to us if we were ill or hurt ourselves. We'd get better, but we couldn't get them from the doctor!

You see, even in the 1970s my gran was a great fan of 'alternative' medicines and standing up for what she believed in. She was a strict vegetarian, campaigned for the disarmament of nuclear weapons on Greenham Common, sabotaged fox hunts (by putting down aniseed to disguise the foxes' scent) and many a time got involved in debates about Scottish currency being legal tender at the checkouts of shops in England (before it was commonly accepted). As kids, we'd look forward to our daily 'medication' of Acerola Plus and screw our faces up in disgust when she tried to get us to drink some revolting brown concoction that came out of a bottle in the fridge. But I did love the visits to the health shop, because it was full of products I didn't see anywhere else, and we seemed to be allowed to top up her basket with far more goodies there than in other shops!

The confidence I took from my gran about being open to non-conventional approaches to healing proved to have a major impact on me in 1991. I'd had a couple of years of experiencing dizziness and blackouts, regularly collapsing at work and ending up in hospital. I went through a whole serious of tests, and had been told I had a 'shadow' on my brain (though not a tumour) before eventually being diagnosed with epilepsy. On one hand, receiving a diagnosis was a relief, but it was also a shock – especially as this meant I lost my driving licence and had to sell the car I'd recently bought. But I accepted the situation and settled into a life of taking lots of tablets each day, as they seemed to work. But after only a few months, I collapsed again while on a skiing holiday with a friend. It transpired that the pharmacist had given me double the strength of tablets I should have had, and I'd unintentionally overdosed on my prescription. Personally, I took my body's reaction as a message that the medication wasn't for me. And this time I chose to listen.

I never touched another tablet for epilepsy and came home from that holiday determined to find another way to take control of my health. Jan De Vries – one of the world's leaders in homeopathy (and a former pharmacist) – happened to have a clinic along the road from my gran in Troon, so I booked an appointment there. In that 1-hour appointment, the homeopath told me he doubted I had epilepsy at all, and thought I'd experienced a rare form of migraine. He gave me a bottle of homeopathic medicine and sent me on my way. I followed his advice and, since finishing the potion he gave me, I've never had any other episodes. Thankfully, my local doctor and hospital consultant had both also experienced the benefits of homeopathy and so, after a few months, were happy to reverse my diagnosis of epilepsy, and I got my driving licence back.

Over twenty years later, and with the knowledge I have, I'm absolutely sure that whatever I was suffering from, I was creating the physical symptoms through the power of my subconscious mind and the mind/body connection. These blackouts were during an unsettling few years emotionally, and while I consciously didn't want to be ill, I now believe that my subconscious mind perceived this as a way for me to get a critical need met until I sorted myself out.

Having since trained in a number of therapies, including Hypnotherapy, Neuro-Linguistic Programming (NLP), and Emotional Freedom Technique (EFT), I've also enjoyed learning the science that supports these complementary approaches. You don't need to be an expert, but having a basic understanding of relevant aspects of science may help you make better-informed decisions about what will work for you. And if you're like me, the science may in fact open your mind to exploring new techniques that will boost your success.

From Wacky to Curiosity

I find it rather odd that modern medicine is deemed to be the best (and only) approach by many, when it's only been around for just over 100 years. Yet other 'natural' or 'alternative' medicines that have been used for hundreds of years (because they work, even though we may not fully understand how – yet) are often classified as 'alternative' and 'incredible'.

Early on in my personal development journey, I used to go to a local Body, Mind & Spirit Fair each summer with one of my good friends. As the years passed, we noticed that what we used to think of as 'a bit odd' had become the norm, and the number of 'whacky' stands at these events seemed to be fewer each year. Despite our different backgrounds (my friend was a director of a pharmaceutical company), we both realised that it was our perceptions and measures of 'wackiness' that had changed, rather than the composition of the events.

In my quest to understand more about how the mind and body works and how we can use this to boost our performance, success and health, I've become particularly curious and excited by new scientific studies exploring the intricate relationship between the heart, brain, body, and Universe we live in. So, let me share some of this with you, as this supports some of the tools I talk about later.

Your Heart is More Than Just a Pump

For decades, medical students in the Western world were taught that the brain is the seat of intelligence and the governor of all things to do with the body, while the purpose of the heart was simply to pump blood around the body. Supported by these conventional beliefs, we've even worked out how to replace an unhealthy heart with the heart of someone who has recently left this physical realm.

However, scientific research now shows that, as well as being one of your body's critical organs, the human heart does far more than just pump blood around the body.

The belief that the heart is more than just a physical organ isn't new. The ancient Egyptians believed it was the heart, rather than the brain, which was the seat of intelligence, thoughts, emotions, and your vital essence. The heart being more than simply a physical organ has been a common thread of spiritual traditions and ancient civilizations.

What is new, is the body of scientific and medical research that has bettered our understanding about the role the heart plays in the way we think, how we feel, the decisions we make, what we do, how we connect with others, and the way we naturally interact with the Universe in which we live.

One of the leading authorities on what is commonly known as Heart Intelligence, is the Institute of HeartMath (IHM) that was set up in 1991 by Doc Childre – a globally recognized, leading authority on reducing stress, building resilience, and optimizing personal effectiveness. Over the last few decades, the team at IHM and many other respected scientists have conducted numerous studies which have challenged previous assumptions about the role and power of the heart.

Let's explore the scope of this incredible resource which is such an integral part of us:

• With very little attention, the human heart usually works for around 70-80 years, beating over 100,000 times a day, pumping over 100 gallons an hour, through a vascular system over sixty thousand miles in length (over twice the circumference of the earth)[5].

• The heart is the first organ formed in a human foetus, and starts to beat before the brain is formed.

• The electromagnetic field of the heart is the strongest produced in the body, and approximately 5000 times more powerful than that of the brain. This field not only permeates every cell in your body, it also extends for up to 10 feet beyond your physical body.[6]

---

5 *The Heartmath Solution, HarperCollins Publishers, Doc Childre & Howard Martin (with Donna Beech),* 2000, Chapter 1, page 9.

6 *The Heartmath Solution, HarperCollins Publishers, Doc Childre & Howard Martin (with Donna Beech),* 2000, Chapter 2, page 33.

- Research conducted in the 1960s and 70s by John and Beatrice Lacey[7] found that there are times when the heart does not obey the signals it receives from the brain. And yet, the brain does obey the signals it receives from the heart. In other words, the heart has the physical ability to influence our thoughts, actions, and behaviours.

- Beating hearts which are removed from the body of someone who is deceased, can continue to beat independently for a period of time even when they are not connected to a brain.

- Since the introduction of human heart transplants, there are an increasing number of studies exploring the numerous reports of heart transplant recipients taking on certain moods, behaviours, knowledge, likes and dislikes of their 'new heart' donor.

The Powerhouse of Your Brain

By comparison, let's acknowledge the supremacy of your brain – the most complex of objects known to man. Weighing approximately three pounds and made up of over 100 billion neurons (nerve cells) [8], this amazing organ is responsible for governing the core functions and maintenance of your body.

I remember growing up with the belief that our brain only grows until a certain age (which I'm sure I've now past!) before dying off cell by cell. And I was so relieved to learn about the advances of science and the ability of the brain to reinvent itself (known as neuroplasticity) through its own activities, and self-directed through the choices that you make; that we can learn new skills (and change the composition of our brains) throughout life; that stroke victims sometimes regain the use of parts of their body previously controlled by a part of the brain that's no longer functioning; and that taking up certain activities (such as learning a new language, style of dance, or musical instrument) can slow down the onset of dementia.

'The science of neuroplasticity shows that each person has the power to change his or her brain for the better. If you don't make use of the power yourself, other forces will shape your

7 Lacey, J., and Lacey, B. Some Autonomic Central Nervous System Interrelationships. In: Black, P., Physi-ological Correlates of Emotion, New York: Academic Press, 1970: 205-227.

8 http://www.alz.org/alzheimers_disease_4719.asp

brain for you, including pressures at work and home, technology and media, pushy people, the lingering effects of painful past experiences and Mother Nature itself.[9]

Rick Hanson, Neuropsychologist & Author

• Until the age of six, children are wandering around in a hypnotic trance – their brains are only operating in 'theta' brain state, which means they are effectively in a hypnotic super-learning brain state (with no conscious filters), recording what's going on around them straight into their subconscious mind.

• The Placebo Effect is a scientifically accepted phenomenon that demonstrates the power your thoughts (and particularly your expectations) have on your physical health – taking placebos (fake drugs) often create biological changes in the body when people believe they are the real drug. In clinical trials for new pharmaceutical drugs, many people often show similar signs of improvement or reduced pain from taking the fake drug rather than the actual drug. To the extent that scientists at reputable medical schools, including Harvard, are exploring how placebos can be used to help people recover from illness – i.e. without taking any pharmaceutical drug.

• The brain uses approximately 25% of the oxygen and nutrients you take into your body to power its continual neural activity (signals between neurons and other parts of your body).

• Your thoughts and feelings change the neural activity in your brain. And your brain influences your thoughts and feelings.

• The neural connections in your brain which have little or no activity wither and die, while those that are most active are 'hardwired' to govern how you respond to what's happening around you. As is often quoted in neuroscience, 'neurons that fire together, wire together'. Hence the benefits of practice and doing more of what makes you feel good to get your desired results!

• It's not uncommon for people to experience phantom pain and sensations in limbs that have been amputated, because of the way the 'body map' in the brain changes post-amputation.[10] Essentially, the 'knowledge' that a person has all four limbs is hardwired, and even post amputation, feelings of that limb can remain.

9 *Hardwiring Happiness, Rick Hanson, The Random House Group, 2013, Chapter 1, p14.*

10 *The Human Mind Documentary, The Documentary Films, YouTube,*

The Relationship Between Your Heart and Brain

Your brain is responsible for many things, including filtering information it receives from the outer world through your senses and past experiences to shape your thoughts and emotions; creating patterns of behaviours; being a store of your memories; analysing and sorting information; releasing chemicals such as hormones in your body; and regulating many of your bodily functions. However, its linear and analytical approach can also have its limitations, particularly if the habits you've developed no longer serve you or if your brain is operating from rigid assumptions.

Your heart, however, is more intuitive in the way it interprets information. By connecting to the positive emotions of love, joy, peace, and compassion in your heart, you'll be more attuned and better able to respond to people and situations in a way that's for your highest good.

Science indicates that there is a two-way communication which continually occurs between the brain and heart. The brain initiates some of this communication, but the heart sends signals to the brain, too, and in four different ways:

- **Neurologically** – sending a burst of neural activity (through the nervous system) from the heart brain with every heartbeat, to parts of the brain that regulate breathing, heart rate, blood vessels, your thinking, perceptions, and other bodily functions.

- **Biochemically** – through the hormonal system, releasing ANF (atrial natriuretic factor) which regulates blood pressure, body-fluid retention, blood vessels, your kidneys, adrenal glands, parts of the brain, inhibits the release of stress hormones, and influences your immune system.

- **Biophysically** – through blood pressure waves pumped around your body.

- **Energetically** – just like a mobile phone mast transmits information outwardly through an electromagnetic field, so does your heart through the strongest electro-magnetic field in the body. It is a field that extends to up to 10 feet outside your body, and can be picked up by those around you.

The Emergence of Heart Intelligence

Since the early 20th century, your IQ (a measure of your ability to read, write, analyse information, apply logic and reasoning) was deemed to be a good indicator of your potential for success. However, in the 1980s, the concept of Emotional Intelligence (EQ) was introduced with the suggestion that our ability to recognise and manage our own emotions, those of others, and to build positive relationships, also influences whether or not we will be successful or perform well.

The numerous scientific studies conducted by the IHM (Institute of Healthcare Management) have expanded our knowledge about the power of the heart, its relationship with the brain, and how – together – they influence how the body works and the way we interact with others. One of their conclusions is that our intelligence and intuition are heightened when we learn to listen more deeply to our heart. And so the phrase Heart Intelligence was born.

The Mind/Body Connection

Some scientists present the view that the mind is a by-product of the brain – that the brain's neural activity creates the mind; and the mind changes the physical structure of the brain. However, Dr Candace Pert (who was pivotal in the discovery of endorphins) suggests another scenario, based on her discovery that molecules of emotion are found all around the body and that 'the mind is not the product of any organ, not even the brain'. Instead, she talked about a 'bodymind' – that cells all through your body collectively form your subconscious mind, storing your memories, experiences, energy and emotional programming.

> *'Molecules of emotion are those of consciousness. Emotions span the material and the immaterial realm: they're the bridge linking the two. Just like the simultaneous particle and wave properties of light, the molecules of emotions go both ways. At the same time, they're physical substances you can see and weigh on a gel in the laboratory, ones that vibrate with an electrical change in the living animal; and they're a kind of physical and psychological, linking brain to body in one vast network of communication to coordinate the entire bodymind.'*[11]

Dr Candice Pert

Wherever the mind 'exists', your thoughts and feelings have an impact on the results you get and the biochemistry of your body.

11 *Everything You Need To Know To Feel Good, Candace B. Pert PHD (with Nancy Marriot), Hay House Publishing, 2007, p45.*

What You Feel Matters

Through their studies, the IHM discovered that when you experience negative emotions such as anger, frustration and stress, the rhythms of your heart appear jagged. Positive emotions such as happiness, love, gratitude and compassion, smooth out the rhythms.

You can see this for yourself by downloading and using IHM 'Emwave' software, which measures your heart-rate variability (heart rhythms) as you experience different emotions. To actually see – on a screen in front of you – your heart rate variability changing immediately in direct correlation to the feelings you choose to feel, is mind-blowing!

But more than that, negative emotions also increase your heart rate; constrict blood vessels; and produce stress hormones such as cortisol and adrenalin. On the other hand, positive emotions slow down your heart rate and blood pressure; release the production of the stress hormone cortisol; increase the production of the anti-aging hormone DHEA; facilitate brain function; and boost the immune system.

So when you focus your attention (your thoughts) on your heart, and choose to experience core emotions such as love, happiness, kindness or compassion, you increase the synchronisation between your heart and brain.

If you want to experience more inner calm and peace (rather than stress, anxiety or worry), it helps to also recognise what's driving what you feel – your head or your heart. Feelings that have conditions, judgement or expectations placed upon them by your thoughts, may tempt you to make decisions or act in a way you later regret. However, when you acknowledge how you feel, take a moment to pause and connect to your heart, you are more likely to take action that will result in a better outcome.

Through the work we do in Rwanda, I've seen first hand how individuals blossom and transform when you give them unconditional love. There is real power in connecting at a heart level before 'trying' to work out how to help, particularly when faced with a distressing or challenging situation. There are times when simply being fully present in the moment and connecting to a feeling of love and compassion in your heart, then doing nothing more than being there and listening, is really powerful for the other person.

If you choose to connect, tap into, and optimise the power of your heart each day, you will improve your health, emotional resilience, relationships, decision-making, and the results you get in all areas of life. And you'll ultimately create a better future for yourself.

I'll be covering the power of emotions and how to manage them for success in more detail in Part 2.

Your Environment Often Matters More Than Your Genes

An old paradigm was that your genes determined how your life was controlled and particularly the traits and propensity to disease that you 'inherited' from your parents. However, as Bruce Lipton explains in his book *The Biology of Belief*, a relatively new field of biology called epigenetics shows that your environment (e.g. nutrition, stress, toxins, and emotions) has a greater impact on your destiny than your genes.

In other words, you have far more scope to influence your physical health and longevity than you may have been led to believe. And you can create the life you want for yourself.

Even the 'Laws' of Physics Change

In 1687, Isaac Newton published his theories of mechanical physics, e.g. the laws of gravity and motion that he proposed applied to all physical matter. However, some of Newton's theories were challenged by 1918 Nobel Prize Winner Max Plank, who discovered that different rules of physics appear to apply at a quantum subatomic level (when studying particles or energy smaller than atoms). Then in 1921, Albert Einstein won a Nobel Prize for developing the theory of relativity (that time and space are relative, not absolute, as Newton had suggested) and for his work towards the development of quantum theory. Today, scientists continue to explore the realms of quantum physics – the invisible energy field that we are all part of and that 'holds' everything in the Universe together; and the role each of us has in creating reality. Our understanding of science is constantly evolving.

What Comes First – Science or Reality?

We are living in a special time, as the wisdom of ancient traditions, spirituality, medical science, and quantum physics come together. At last science is beginning to explain why and how many of the traditional customs which have been practised for thousands of years (e.g. meditation and prayer), are of benefit to us as individuals, to society, and to the world. We are learning how we can optimise our incredible bodies within the galactic Universe to help shape the life we'd love to create for ourselves.

In her book, *Dying To Be Me*, Anita Moorjani[12] shares the remarkable story of her recovery from cancer, which has been documented by oncologists across the world. She openly admits she doesn't know why she had the opportunity to recover when others don't, and doesn't make any claims about how to cure cancer. However, what she does recount is her personal experience and what she attributes to her unbelievably speedy recovery when, according to the medics around her, she 'should' be dead. The pivotal factor in her view was the feeling of unconditional love (being free of judgment and other head-driven emotions) that she experienced while her cancer-ridden body was shutting down. While this hasn't been 'proven' yet, there are many studies exploring the phenomenon of near-death experiences, and how miraculous recoveries from physical illnesses and injuries do occur.

I used to be a sceptic about anything that wasn't scientifically proven. But I now realise that science is often actually about providing rationale and understanding for what is first experienced and seen, but cannot be explained. And also, that scientific 'evidence' is usually decades behind what we, as humans, experience and seek cures for.

Think about it. In order for the findings of any scientific study to be taken seriously by many 'Western' minds, there is a lengthy process which scientists need to go through. This often involves observing what's happening (not just one-offs, but a sequence of reported and unexplained 'miracles'), getting buy-in (and funding) to conduct a thorough research project, conducting the research (which in itself could take years), evaluating the research, and then publishing the findings.

For something to be proven scientifically, it usually requires an identified pattern or sequence of events to yield a predictable result, over a period of time, in a controlled and monitored setting.

Sometimes it can be the results of research or exploratory procedures that change beliefs around what's possible. This has been demonstrated by the pioneering work of UK scientists and Polish surgeons who have just published a report on how they have enabled a formerly paralysed man to walk again, opening up renewed hope for millions of paralysed people around the world.[13]

---

12 *Dying To Be Me, Anita Moorjani, Hay House Publishing, 2012*

13 *http://www.bbc.co.uk/news/health-29645760*

Thankfully, there are many in the science and medical communities who, through their open-mindedness and curiosity, are questioning some of the beliefs and limitations of conventional science and are offering us a more holistic perspective on how we work – as human beings and as the mass of energy we are, within the greater galactic universe. Unfolding secrets to our survival that are as ground-breaking as the discovery that the world is round not flat!

You are an incredible being with so much untapped potential – are you ready to experience what your body, mind and spirit wants to help you achieve?

Recommended Resources

- *Everything You Need To Know To Feel Good* by Candace B. Pert

- *The HeartMath Solution* by Doc Childre & Howard Martin (with Donna Beech)

- HeartMath – http://www.heartmath.com/

- *Hardwiring Happiness* by Rick Hanson

- *The Human Mind* by Professor Robert Winston

- *Dying To Be Me* by Anita Moorjani

PART 2

- The 9 Principles of Heart-Centered Success -

Chapter 4

Principle 1 – Engage Your Heart

In all you do – towards yourself, the way you connect with others, and respond to situations.

'Despite everything, I believe that people are really good at heart.'
Anne Frank, Author & Genocide Victim

Isn't that an incredibly poignant quote from Anne Frank? Whenever I read this, it brings tears to my eyes and I feel a tug in my heart knowing she subsequently died, aged only 15, in one of the Nazi concentration camps during the Second World War. Those who commit atrocities like this don't seem to 'engage their hearts' in the way most of us do.

This principle is about engaging your heart and inviting the purest form of your inner being to guide the way you treat yourself, treat others, respond to situations, and decide what to do, by applying the following values in your approach:

- **Love** – be the embodiment of love. Listen and be true to the guidance of your heart.

- **Kindness** – act with kindness and generosity.

- **Compassion** – connect with how all living creatures feel, and then take action to eliminate suffering.

- **Integrity** – be true and authentic to the pure essence of who you were born to be.

- **Respect** – treat yourself with respect, be mindful of and honour rights and opinions of others.

- **Gratitude** – be appreciative and express gratitude.

- **Peace** – release the past, be forgiving, and let go of future worries.

When you embrace these values, you appreciate the beauty of who you are inside; you feel good about yourself; you accept that you always do the best you can; you look after your health; you align how you spend your time to what will nourish your soul. You're also more likely to be successful in achieving your desired results and to respond more calmly and effectively to challenging situations.

As I mentioned in the previous chapter, science shows that coming from a place of love, kindness, compassion, forgiveness, and gratitude, helps you to be healthier and increase your propensity to live longer, too.

Let me ask you a question – do any of the following make you feel really good (in the moment or in the long-term)?

- embracing self-criticism or self-sabotage

- not honouring your personal needs

- allowing others to treat you badly

- overeating or drinking to excess

- not exercising enough

- not being true to yourself or others

Most people experiencing any of these are not jumping around with energy and joy! Rather, these behaviours are all indicators of an opportunity for change – so that you feel better and get better results. It is far more enjoyable to engage your heart, and to treat yourself in the way an educated, loving parent would treat their child.

Some people view self-love or appreciation as self-indulgence, but – just as parents on an airplane are asked to fit their own oxygen masks before those of their children – you need to nurture yourself in order to be the best support you can be to others.

And you just don't know the impact your heartfelt actions will have on the lives of others, as is demonstrated by this true story, which I share with kind permission from Martin Stepek:

Sixth of December 1941. Somewhere in Siberia. It's cold, dark, and the snow is feet thick.

On a cattle truck, stuck in a railway siding, hundreds of exhausted Poles are crammed, hungry and ill. They have recently been freed from the dreaded Siberian gulags and are seeking to flee the Soviet Union, but they have few resources, and their energy is spent.

Four of the refugees are dear to me. My father is one. He is 19 years old. His two sisters, Zosia and Danka, are 16 and 14, and their mother, Janina, is 39. She has been unable to get up for three months now, desperately sick, worn out, and starving. The family haven't eaten for a week, and are surviving by melting the snow on the ground and the icicles that form all day long on their cattle train.

Then another train, filled with Russians fleeing the advancing German forces, stops on the next track. All of the Polish refugees, aching with hunger, start to beg from the Russian people on the other train, and the Russians generously share some of their food with them.

Little Danka is watching this from the opened grille, which serves as the carriage window. Jan and Zosia have been out begging, leaving her to tend to her mother. They return empty-handed and are desolate. Danka hears the word 'Divotchka' amongst the bustle of Polish beggars and Russian givers. Again she hears it: 'Divotchka.' It means little girl. She starts looking for the source. A Russian woman, wrapped in a thick fur coat and hat, is standing at the door of the other train. Danka stares at her. The woman is young and beautiful, maybe thirty years old. She stares back and smiles at the girl. Then she delves into the bag at her side and she throws something large and heavy straight at Danka. Instinctively, Danka ducks but catches it. It is a huge loaf of bread. She looks up to thank the lady but she is gone.

This loaf feeds the family for a week. Without it, they would all have died of hunger. The date was sixth of December, St Nicholas's day. It is the day Polish children receive their presents.

I can never know who this woman was who saved my father and his two sisters, and prolonged the life of my grandmother so that when she finally died of hunger, she did so knowing that her children were free from the Soviet Union. Several other strangers, many of them impoverished Muslim peasant farmers in Uzbekistan and Kazakhstan, shared what little they had to help my father and his family. It is due to their altruism that I came to have a life, and in turn now have my own two children. My nine brothers and sisters, and our children, all owe our lives to these unknown people. Of all human traits it is this, the kindness of strangers in the most trying of times, which I think is most astonishing and moving, and it is our great source of hope.

One of the great pleasures in life is to do something kind with no expectation.

Obviously, your intentions and actions only have a part to play in what you experience, because there are many factors you can't control, including how others respond to you. In every situation, the best you can be is to act with positive intention and love in your heart, while at the same time accepting you are doing the best you can. In other words, to focus on being the best version of yourself.

In terms of success, you are far more likely to succeed at things which engage and touch your heart – the things that excite you, motivate you, compel you to take action, which add meaning to your life, or make you feel warm inside.

• Do you remember a goal that you were really pleased to achieve? What motivated you to achieve it? What were the benefits to you of achieving this goal?

• By comparison, think of a goal you consciously wanted to achieve but didn't because – if you're totally honest – something inside held you back?

In the next few chapters we'll be exploring each of these intrinsically linked heart values in more detail.

As with applying all the principles, the most important aspect to remember is to apply these first towards yourself, then towards others and situations you are facing.

Occasionally, clients have asked me to help them change how someone else is treating them, but one of the first things I explain is that we cannot control what others do (or don't do). However, you can change what you think, feel, do, and how you act, so that you become more influential in your interactions with others. In other words, when you change, you *may* find others change, too.

When you become aware of your thought patterns, emotional triggers and behaviours, you can heal and change what is sabotaging the results you are getting. Once you've done this, you'll often be very pleasantly surprised to find that your interactions with others are easier and more effective. You may also experience fewer challenges and instead be presented with opportunities that reflect what you're looking for.

By contrast, trying to change someone else or overcome challenges without considering the part you are playing in creating the situation, is often a strategy for frustration, stress and disappointment.

In the following chapters, I therefore focus on explaining how to apply the heart values towards yourself first, and also share ideas for applying them towards others.

Chapter 5

Principle 1 – Heart Value – Love

Be the embodiment of love towards yourself and others. Listen and be true to the inner guidance of your heart.

I love the opening scenes of the film '*Love Actually*'. It warms my heart to be reminded that, despite what we hear through the media every day about what's wrong in the world, love is all around us if we just take the time to notice. And there's no better place to witness it than at the Arrivals hall in any airport. There, you find people eagerly waiting for loved ones to appear, watching the doors with anticipation and love in their hearts. Then, when they first catch sight of their loved ones, a smile instinctively breaks out and they feel good inside. When they meet, a hug or a kiss are the most natural expressions of love and affection.

If you take the time to pause from the hectic pace of life and look about, you will see love all around you, too – parents exchanging tender moments with their children; couples holding hands; the laughter of children playing and having fun; someone cuddling a dog or stroking a cat; people gazing fondly at a baby in a pram.

Obviously, whether you feel these special moments as love or not when you observe them, will depend on where you are emotionally. If you've recently lost someone close to you, you may feel a sense of loss or sadness in response to the sight of others enjoying love. And it's perfectly natural to feel that way, though there are ways to help you accelerate your own healing.

Love is one of the most precious gifts of life that we can give to ourselves; and to others. It is an essential ingredient for a happy and healthy life; it helps you feel alive; it adds meaning and purpose to life.

'Love is your original energy. It's the heart of who you are.'

Robert Holden, Author

Each and every one of us was born into this world with the same rights, including the right to love and feel loved. However, sometimes our ability to feel loved can be tainted by the critical opinions or unkind actions of others towards us. And this in turn can restrict our perceived ability to love unconditionally. Again, there are ways to heal ourselves from any hurt we experience in life, which I'll come on to shortly.

Love is the natural essence and spirit of who you are – the way you were when you were born and, depending on your belief systems, continue to 'be' after we leave the physical world. Your natural state is one of love. It's the purest part of you that is free of any self-criticism or judgment. The energy of love is inside you, as well as being all around you. Many people seek love from those around them, but love is an emotion you can feel inside without the need to get this from others.

The first step towards enjoying a life of love, is to embrace self-love. It's only once you love yourself that you'll enjoy the experience of love in its true unconditional form.

When you were born, you were free of any self-criticism or doubt: these are things you've learned and chosen to believe to be true, because of your life experiences. Remember, until the age of around seven, you were wandering through life in a super-hypnotic learning state, with no conscious filters to make sense of the information you were exposed to. Many of the beliefs you now have about yourself and love will be recordings of what those around you taught you when you were young, and which you stored in your unconscious mind. These unconscious beliefs are influencing what you experience as an adult, because your thoughts and feelings drive your actions and how you respond to situations around you. So, unless you've proactively detoxed your mind as an adult, your experience today is based upon what you learned to be true as a child.

If most of the messages you heard when you were young were expressions of unconditional love and acceptance from those around you, such as the words 'I love you' and physical acts of affection, then you are more likely to love and accept yourself as an adult and to experience healthy loving relationships with others. However, if your experiences of love when you were young were neglect, fuelled with anger or physical abuse, you're likely to think, feel, and act very differently. You may not like yourself, and doubt whether you are good enough. Or you may feel rejected, have difficulties in trusting others, or forming healthy relationships. Many people who've not felt loved when growing up, find it hard to express love in a healthy way as an adult.

If you don't feel you love yourself, don't worry. In the same way you have learned to think and feel the way you do today, you can learn how to think and feel differently about yourself: if you want to. Whatever your experiences have been, you can learn to be more loving towards yourself from today. By choosing to heal with self-love, you'll put yourself in a much better place emotionally to attract a healthy uplifting form of love, contentment, and success in your life.

I feel very fortunate to recently have been introduced to an incredible guy called Brett. My conversations with him are both enthralling and inspiring; they always bring a smile to my face. What is most refreshing is his enthusiasm for life and his overt expressions of love. He's like a young puppy, with boundless energy and unconditional love for all around – his charisma is infectious. His words and what he's doing in life today are clearly reflections of the limitless love, kindness, and compassion in his heart. This grown man has learned to love and accept himself for the true essence of love that he is, and this is reflected in the people he now has around him in his life. But it hasn't always been that way. Seeking the love of his dad, he found himself living a life of crime. And while he knew in his heart what he was doing wasn't 'right' and he had more to offer, he found himself addicted to drugs and serving time in prison. Many in that situation would believe that was their destiny, but for Brett the birth of his daughter was the catalyst for change – he embarked upon a personal journey of transformation, appeared in a ground-breaking film, and has helped many disadvantaged young people in the UK and Africa. By choosing to take the leap of faith that he did, Brett has created a life of joy, love, and passion, and his abundant heart-felt energy is infectious.[14]

You, too, can enjoy success when you engage your heart.

Take a moment to consider what you've learned about love:

---

14 You can find out more about Brett's transformational journey by watching the film Choice Point or by reading the book of the same title by Harry Massey & Dr David Hamilton.

- What do you remember being told about yourself when you were young?

- How did you experience love as a young child?

- How has this shaped how you feel about yourself?

- What did you learn about how to express love?

- How has this influenced how you express love as an adult?

When we love ourselves, we feel connected to the true essence of who we are and feel peace inside; we see past the physical face reflected in the mirror, and love the spirit smiling back at us through our eyes; we accept we always do the best we can, even when we need to find peace in our hearts and forgive ourselves for something we've done; we let go of any of the doubts or critical thoughts we've learned about ourselves during our journey through life; we accept compliments rather than throwing them back at the person who's expressed them (like a slap to their face); we don't over-indulge our bodies with food, drink or other toxic substances; and we don't consider or carry out acts of jealousy, retaliation, aggression or neglect: these are expressions of a lack of love – for self and others.

What you feel about yourself has a direct impact on how you love and experience love from others. When we love and accept ourselves, our experience of love in relationships is greatly enriched and very different from entering into a relationship with a desperate 'need' to be liked or loved by someone else to make us feel good. I remember someone once saying to me – if you don't love yourself, how can you possibly expect others to love you and treat you well? And they were absolutely right. When we love and respect ourselves, we don't feel insecure or allow others to hurt or mistreat us. Rather, our experience of relationships will be one of love, joy, nourishment and strength – both in terms of what we give out and what we receive.

Whether you love yourself or not will also have a huge impact on the type of success you'll experience in all areas of life.

You attract people and opportunities that resonate with the person and energy you project. If you doubt or dislike yourself, this will be reflected in what you say, how you act, and what you do. And you'll attract others who are looking to connect with people who feel this way about themselves. However, when you focus on being the wonderful and unique person you were born to be, and do what it takes to feel really confident to step out into the world as this, you will attract others into your life who love and value the confident, unique you.

Once you love and embrace your best authentic self, focus on doing what you love, and are good at and connect with others with love in your heart, beautiful miracles start to unfold. You will feel good about yourself and be able to project this with confidence.

A good starting point is to recognise how you feel about yourself today. To do this, simply say the following statement aloud and rate how true it feels to you, on a scale of 0-10 (with 10 being absolutely true; and 0 being 'I don't feel this way at all'):

'I deeply and completely accept myself, love myself and forgive myself.'

If you're able to say this aloud and honestly feel this as being true, you're well on your way to opening your heart to the joys of love.

If this doesn't feel true to you yet, please don't worry. Many people don't feel this way about themselves. A lower score simply indicates that there is lots of scope for you to learn how to feel better about yourself.

Ways to Enjoy More Love

It's possible for you to learn to experience more love and success if you want it. Here are some very simple ways you can immediately start to nurture a great sense of self-love:

- **The Mirror Technique**

  One of the first techniques I learned to feel better about myself was from Louise Hay in her book, You Can Heal Your Life. Initially it seemed really silly and odd, but because what I'd been doing until then wasn't making me feel happy inside, I decided to give it a try, no matter how daft it felt. It was great to then discover that it really does work; just laughing at myself in the moment changed how I felt.

  When you look at yourself in the mirror, what do you say to yourself? Are you nourishing your heart with love by saying to yourself, 'I love you', 'you are great', or 'you are wonderful'? Or are you more likely to be being unkind to yourself by thinking negative thoughts, such as, 'you're fat', 'you're ugly', or 'I hate you'?

  If you haven't done this before, I encourage you to go and look at yourself in the mirror now. Then:

1. Notice what you're thinking as you look at your reflection in the mirror.

2. Smile at your reflection and tell the face smiling back, 'I love and accept you as you are' and other terms of endearment you might say to a young child whom you love unconditionally.

3. Be aware of (and note down) how you feel about saying this, and particularly any negative thoughts and feelings, so that you can take action to turn these around (e.g. using affirmations (Chapter 21) or tapping (Chapter 22)).

4. Please be reassured, too, that many people find this a very challenging and emotional exercise to do. So if you feel you are unable to do this yet, be kind to yourself. There are ways you can heal whatever is holding you back from feeling this way about yourself.

- **Mind Detox**

One of the great disciplines I learned when I first studied EFT was the Personal Peace Procedure. This involves noting down all the negative emotions and beliefs you experience. Then diligently work through these to eliminate what isn't working, and replace them with thoughts and feelings that will support you in becoming the best version of yourself. It's a great way to clear your emotional and mental baggage.

A very simple way of doing this is to write 'I am...' on a piece of paper, and write down whatever word(s) first comes to mind. Keep saying 'I am' and trust your unconscious to continue to finish off the sentence with what you think and feel about yourself. You could ask your unconscious mind to focus on positive beliefs first, then move on to the negative, or vice versa. Or you can simply list whatever comes up and then highlight the positive and negative.

If you find it hard to come up with a list yourself, check out the link at the end of this chapter, where you can download the Heart-Centered Success Questionnaire. It contains a list of many statements that will enable you to identify what thoughts and feelings you have that are contributing to the results you are currently getting.

Once you have done this, congratulate yourself on all the positive beliefs and feelings that you have about yourself! And learn to turn around negative beliefs and feelings you've identified, using a whole range of techniques, including affirmations and tapping that I cover in more detail in Chapter 15 – Manage Your Thoughts & Emotions.

- **Collect Compliments**

  How do you feel when someone gives you a compliment? Many people have become masters at shrugging off compliments, yet at the same time holding on tightly to comments they find hurtful or upsetting. I used to do the same until someone suggested that shrugging off a compliment is like slapping someone in the face and telling them they're talking rubbish! I had never thought before that shrugging off a compliment is rude and disrespectful to the other person. But when you do this, you're not respecting their opinion. Surely if someone has taken the time so share what they think, it's more polite to say 'thank you'. And remember to jot the compliment down in your Success Journal (whether or not you believe it to be true), so you can refer to it at any time you need a boost to how you feel about yourself.

You will discover more techniques to nourish your heart in forthcoming chapters, as many of the heart values and nine principles are interlinked.

Simple Ways to Demonstrate Love Towards Others

- Tell them you love them (as long as you do)!

- Demonstrate love to others in the way they recognise love, rather than the way you like love to be expressed.

  Many people treat others in a way that they themselves like to be treated, which is a great starting point. But, sometimes expressions of love can be missed or misinterpreted simply because there are different ways to express love. In his book, *The Five Love Languages*, Gary Chapman explains that we express our love in different ways – quality time; words of affirmation; gifts; acts of service; physical touch.

  You may like spending time with your partner, but they may express their love by buying you presents. Or, they may like doing things for you, but you'd prefer them to tell you how much they love you.

  Having been through a divorce, where a lack of effective communication was a contributing factor, I was eager to make sure this didn't happen again. So, early on in my relationship with my second husband, we had a discussion about our primary love languages. Bless him for 'playing along' when I'm sure he would have preferred to 'keep it simple', but I honestly do think that understanding what's important for each of us has helped us enjoy an incredibly harmonious relationship where we both feel valued and loved for who we are.

- With children, spend time with them doing what they want to do (e.g. playing a game they love, watching the film they want to watch, doing an activity they enjoy) rather than how you'd prefer to spend time with them.

- When someone hurts or upsets you, release these negative feelings (see Chapter 15) so you can approach the person or situation with feelings of love, kindness, and compassion in your heart.

Resourceful Questions

Be really honest and ask yourself the following questions to give you ideas how you could experience more love:

- How could I be more loving towards myself?

- How could I be more loving towards others?

- What do I love about life?

- What do I love to do?

- How could I bring more love into my life?

Empowering Affirmations to Nurture Your Heart

- I always do the best I can.

- I love and accept myself the way I am.

- I deserve to be loved.

- I deserve to be happy.

- I release the past and forgive everyone.

Tapping 'Set Up' Statements

- Even though I find it hard to love myself, I deeply and completely accept myself.

- Even though I don't feel good enough, I accept I always do the best I can.

- Even though I don't feel loved, I know I deserve to be loved.

Recommended Resources

- *You Can Heal Your Life* by Louise Hay
- *I Heart Me, The Science Of Self Love* by Dr David R. Hamilton
- *Loveability: Knowing How To Love And Be Loved* by Dr Robert Holden
- *The Five Love Languages* by Gary Chapman
- *Zest for Life* by Dawn Breslin
- *Choice Point* – the film and book (by Harry Massey & Dr David R. Hamilton)

Chapter 6

Principle 1 – Heart Value – Kindness

Act with kindness and generosity towards yourself and others.

Did you know that kindness is good for your physical health, your emotional wellbeing, and makes you more attractive to others? Mind Body Scientist and author Dr David Hamilton shares many studies on this topic in his book, *Why Kindness Is Good For You.*

Put simply, the act of being kind releases a range of natural feel-good hormones in your body, including oxytocin and endorphins. So practising kindness, compassion, and appreciation can make you happier, boost your immune system, reverse the signs of aging, relieve pain, and even help you live longer. Choosing to think and feel kindness about someone you find challenging, ahead of interacting or responding to them, is one of my favourite strategies for changing how I feel in the moment (e.g. releasing stress or anxiety), and is an excellent strategy for defusing potentially difficult situations.

Human beings are genetically wired to be kind. Kindness comes from our ability as a species to relate to one another, feel empathy and compassion towards one another, and the desire we naturally have to eliminate suffering and help each other. Being kind and generous on an unconditional basis is a natural and effective way to connect with others.

'The best part of life is not just surviving, but thriving with passion and compassion and humour and style and generosity and kindness.'

Maya Angelou, Author & Poet

True acts of kindness are made without any attachment or expectation to an outcome; they are what you feel compelled to do as a loving and caring human being. Studies show that being kind towards others is a highly effective way to change how you feel and even reduce feelings of depression, because it requires focusing on someone other than yourself.

And often the acts of kindness that are most appreciated are the small yet important things which you may never know the outcome of.

I was at an event recently and, during an interval, I went to the toilet. As I was walking towards a cubicle that was being vacated, the woman who came out offered me a tissue from her handbag as there was no toilet paper. And, on hearing this exchange, the woman in the next cubicle passed through a roll of toilet paper. If you've ever gone into a public toilet only to realise too late that there's a lack of toilet paper, you'll know how much you'd appreciate such gestures!

In business I'm often very pleasantly surprised by the ever flowing, spontaneous acts of kindness and generosity of those I've connected with. Often what may have seemed like a small thing to them has transformed my business in terms of scope, impact, and financial rewards. I've been personally introduced to many people who have given me business, or helped me out; through discussion, they've enabled me to work towards greater goals; they've been generous with their time and, in many instances, they have become great friends. Without doubt, my business would not have succeeded without the generosity of others. And I always aim to be that way with people, too.

Have you noticed that some people ooze kindness, while others just don't seem to think of others? Like many of our behaviours, the way we express kindness is greatly influenced by what we experienced when we were growing up. What did you learn from your parents and those around you about being kind? I have friends who learned from their parents to put kindness as a human quality above most other 'measures of success' in life; that being kind and loving was the most important thing in life. Whereas others were taught to place greater importance on academic, career, or sporting achievements. There is no right or wrong, but what we learned about kindness when we were young undoubtedly shapes who we become, what we naturally feel inclined to do, and how we engage in life.

Most of us have learned that kindness is a desirable human behaviour. Yet some people receive conflicting messages between what they were 'told' and the behaviours they experienced or observed. I'm sure you'll have met some people who come across as being kind but then their actions conflict with their words. They may perceive themselves as being kind, but go around hurting or abusing others. If you're honest with yourself, has there ever been a time when you have been unkind to someone?

You are more likely to engage in spontaneous acts of kindness when you're fully present in the moment and not distracted by other more pressing things on your mind. Think about it: when you're running around with lots on your mind, do you ever get to your destination with very little awareness about the people you passed along your way? If this is the case, is there any scope that you'll have missed an opportunity to be kind to someone? To stop and help an elderly person across the street; to notice and pick up a glove a young child has dropped; to listen and respond with kindness to what's being said or not said?

As well as being present in the moment to respond to day-to-day events which give you the opportunity to be kind, consciously setting the intention to be kind to someone each day or in a particular situation can also change how you feel and make a difference to others. You could even find that, as a result, others around you change, more opportunities present themselves, and you experience unexpected benefits.

'When we feel love and kindness toward others, it not only makes others feel loved and cared for, but it helps us also to develop inner happiness and peace.'

His Holiness, The 14th Dalai Lama [15]

You may have heard of the book or film, Pay It Forward. It's an inspiring story about a 12-year-old boy who is challenged by a social studies teacher to 'think of an idea for world change and put it into action'. His idea is to do something good for three people and to ask them to 'pay it forward', so that collectively they create a human wave of kindness. On the back of the film, The Pay It Forward movement was born. The idea is that you do a good deed for someone else, without expecting anything in return other than that they 'pay it forward' to someone else. To proactively come up with an idea in

---

15 *The Kindness Foundation - http://www.randomactsofkindness.org*

advance and do it. Or when you're faced with an opportunity, to do this in the course of a day. There is no such thing as too small an act of kindness.

It's also worth being aware of how acts of kindness trigger certain behaviours – in yourself and others. In his book, Influence; The Psychology Of Persuasion, Robert Cialdini talks about the principle of 'reciprocity' that relates to how we human beings have a tendency to feel the need to reciprocate or respond favourably to requests made by people we perceive as having done something for us.

If I give an example, a few years ago I decided to learn how to play golf. My golf instructor had very kindly lent me a club I could use to practise my swing at home and at the driving range, until I decided whether I wanted to invest in a set of clubs. After a few weeks of really enjoying my lessons (and apparently making surprisingly good progress), I thought it was time to buy my own clubs. I did some research on eBay and decided I'd ask my instructor for his advice. Knowing all about the principle of 'reciprocity' (and how this is a major influencing factor for me when making buying decisions), I went to my next lesson with the intention of only asking for advice and with the specific intention that I'd say 'no' to any clubs he may have.

I was delighted that he agreed it was time for me to get a full set of clubs, and he gave me some really useful tips about what to buy. Then I found myself with a bit of a dilemma: he'd had a client trade in her first set that week. He could offer them to me for £50 just now, and would happily buy them back from me when I was ready to trade up. So here was what was going through my mind: he's lent me his club for the last six weeks, and now he's offering me a deal that in the long-term isn't going to cost me a penny. He's been kind to me once and now is being kind again – how can I say no?

While one factor that led me to buy those clubs was the low financial cost, the main driver was that the thought of saying 'no' and holding onto the club he'd lent me now seemed selfish. And I didn't want to be perceived as being selfish. My instructor's act of kindness in lending me the club resulted in me going home that day with the clubs in the boot of my car, laughing to myself at what had just happened.

The reason I highlight this is that, by being human, you are being influenced all the time by others' acts of kindness – so it is in your interest to know what is influencing you. Have you ever been compelled to take certain action because the other person had previously been kind or done you a favour?

Likewise, you are influencing the decisions of others by being kind, in terms of how they are likely to respond to you and any requests you make of them. While I'm an advocate of unconditional acts of love, kindness, and compassion, it is important to recognise when setting personal boundaries could be in the highest interests of you and others.

If you want to experience more kindness in your life, the first step is to be more kind to yourself. I meet lots of very thoughtful, kind and generous people, who are precious pearls in their community. But many forget to be kind to themselves as well, and often end up feeling knackered, ill, and frustrated, because they are not getting their personal needs met. Sometimes this goes on to result in feelings of resentment and depression. Giving to others at the expense of what you need yourself, is not sustainable, whereas being kind to yourself gives you greater capacity to be kind to others.

As Mahatma Gandhi once said, 'Be the change that you wish to see in the world.'[16] In other words, if you want to experience success, confidence, happiness, or any of the heart values, you first need to feel and live them yourself. Then, notice how others respond to you and the opportunities that present themselves.

Ways to Be More Kind

• Kindness Challenge

Commit to consciously being kind to yourself and others, with a random act of kindness. Being kind to yourself could include time for yourself, what you eat or drink, and what you expose yourself to. There are so many ways you can be kind to others.

You could make this more fun and impactful by involving others in your challenge. Remember to note what you do and how you're feeling in your Success Journal (Introduction Chapter). A great resource for ideas is The Random Acts Of Kindness Foundation (www.therandomactsofkindnessfoundation.org). You don't have to think about exactly how you will be kind – by simply setting this intention and being present in the moment as you go about your day, opportunities will arise.

16 https://www.goodreads.com/quotes/24499-be-the-change-that-you-wish-to-see-in-the

• Kindness Blast

One of the easiest and most effective ways to let go of negative emotions you feel in relation to a challenging person (such as stress, anxiety, hurt, upset or anger), is to 'send' them kindness.

I recently worked with a business owner who was tempted to post angry comments on Facebook about a supplier who had let her down. But she decided to neutralise her frustration by imagining sending them 'love, kindness, and compassion' instead. Taking the time to do this put her in a better emotional place and she chose a more effective response – to write a private email. By doing this, she quickly felt better and saved a lot of time and energy. She also avoided potential reputational damage.

To 'send kindness':

1. Think of someone or something you feel overwhelming love and compassion towards.
2. Notice how when you do this, you start to feel love and compassion in your heart.
3. As you continue to think of them, connect the feeling of kindness in your heart. Imagine this feeling in your heart having a colour – if it did, what colour would it be?
4. Imagine filling your body with this colourful feeling of love, kindness, and compassion.
5. Now imagine sending this feeling from your heart to the person or situation that is challenging you, in whatever way your unconscious mind wants to do this. Just trust what comes up.
6. Continue to hold and send this feeling for a few minutes.
7. Notice how you feel when you're doing this.
8. Once you've finished, notice how differently you feel towards the person or situation.
9. Then ask yourself how you could respond effectively to the situation.

Sometimes it can also be helpful to first do some tapping to let go of the negative emotion.

Resourceful Questions

Be really honest and ask yourself the following questions to give you ideas how you could experience more kindness:

- How could I be more kind towards myself?

- How could I be more kind towards others?

- What could I do differently each day to have more opportunities to be kind?

Empowering Affirmations To Nurture Your Heart

- I am a kind and loving person.

- I deserve to be treated with love, kindness, and compassion.

- The more kind I am to myself, the better I feel.

- The more kind I am towards others, the better I feel.

Tapping 'Set Up' Statements

- Even though I find it hard to be kind to myself, I deeply and completely accept I always do the best I can.

- Even though I find it easier to be kinder to others than myself, I deeply and completely love and accept myself.

- Even though I feel others don't treat me with love and kindness, I know I can start by being kind to myself.

Recommended Resources

- *Why Kindness Is Good For You* by Dr David R. Hamilton

- The Random Acts Of Kindness Foundation (www.therandomactsofkindnessfoundation.org)

Chapter 7

Principle 1 – Heart Value – Compassion

Connect with how all living creatures feel, and take action to eliminate suffering.

Did you know that being compassionate helps to reduce your risk of heart disease?

Research conducted by Dacher Keltner (Professor of Psychology at University of Berkley) suggests that practicing compassion slows down your heart rate[17] and produces the hormone oxytocin (which, among other benefits, boosts your immune system, softens your arteries, reduces blood pressure, reduces inflammation, and aids digestion).

Recent advances in science and technology also show that being compassionate enhances emotional and physical wellbeing; helps to make us feel good; is a powerful antidote for personal healing; helps to create harmonious relationships; engenders a more positive and optimistic approach to life; and makes it easier to cope with life's challenges.

Someone who demonstrates compassion is also often considered to be trustworthy, which is a key component of whether people will be friendly, work with you, work for you, spend time around you, or buy from you. So your ability to feel and demonstrate compassion will influence your success in all areas of life.

The practice of developing compassion as a skill has existed in many Eastern traditions for hundreds of years and, having been the focus of many studies, is now becoming increasingly recognized as an important aspect of emotional wellbeing, resilience, and performance in Western cultures, too.

---

17 *http://greatergood.berkeley.edu/topic/compassion/definition#what_is*

Professor Paul Gilbert defines compassion as 'a basic kindness, with a deep awareness of the suffering of oneself and other living things, coupled with the wish and effort to relieve it'.[18]

During a talk at Stanford University in October 2010, the Dalai Lama referred to how families living in a compassionate home are much happier than those who have money without compassion, love, affection, and trust.[19] Tibetan monks consider compassion as more than just an emotion – that it is a natural force or energy that connects everything in the Universe.[20]

There is a subtle distinction between feeling compassion and feeling sympathy towards someone. When we associate with how the other person feels and get drawn into the suffering ourselves, this feeling is sympathy. By contrast, demonstrating compassion is about relating to the other person's suffering and taking action to help eliminate it.

It is our ability to feel love, compassion, and our motivation to eliminate others' suffering that often triggers acts of kindness. That may involve doing something to make the situation better for them. Other times, it could simply be about being fully present in the moment, with love in our hearts, and holding the space for them to move through their suffering.

We have an endless supply of compassion within us, despite what is sometimes referred to as 'compassion fatigue'. Think of the last time you saw footage of a natural disaster or war on TV, and especially the images of young children and injured innocent people caught up in a horrific situation. When you saw this type of scene, did your heart 'go out' to these people?

In the UK we have a charity called Children In Need which is making a difference to the lives of many children around the world. Each year the whole country comes together through schools, workplaces, community projects and national initiatives, to raise money for the projects they support. Part of this event is an evening of entertainment and film coverage of the individuals and groups the charity has helped. It's our ability to feel compassion that leads many people, including grown men and woman of all ages, to have tears in their eyes at numerous points throughout this programme. And it is our capacity to feel compassion that compels us to put

18 *The Compassionate Mind, Paul Gilbert, Constable & Robinson, 2010, Introduction, pxii*

19 *https://www.youtube.com/watch?v=uSL_xvokoF8&index=1&list=PL3A1585C4EDE6E82D*

20 *The Divine Matrix, Gregg Braden, Hay House, 2007, p85*

our hands in our pockets to support this and other charities.

We live in a world where anger, frustration, and hatred threaten our survival, that of many species, and the sustainability of the planet. However, when we replace destructive feelings of anger, resentment, fear, judgment, and hatred with empathy, love, and compassion, we stand a much better chance of co-creating a more peaceful world for ourselves, those we care about, and the global community of which we are a part.

This is one of the reasons that we help genocide survivors in Rwanda to feel compassion and forgiveness for those who committed the most heinous crimes against them, their families, and their communities. Finding peace in their hearts is part of the healing process they undergo on a personal level, so that collectively they can create a more harmonious future for their country. The aim is a more compassionate, progressive, and sustainable alternative to civil war or terrorism.

When you choose to embrace love and compassion, you recognise that everyone (including yourself and those who hurt you) always does the best they can. And that those who 'hurt' us, are often suffering in some way themselves.

Our ability to feel compassion is linked to our ability to feel peace, acceptance, and forgiveness in our heart, and to act in alignment with these heart values. One of the most incredible stories of compassion and forgiveness is that of Immaculee Ilibagiza as recounted in her book, *Left To Tell.*

During the Rwandan genocide, Immaculee's family was brutally murdered by many former friends. Her survival was down to the kind and brave acts of a local pastor who hid her and seven other Tutsi women in an en-suite shower room, behind a wardrobe, for 90 days. While in hiding, Immaculee could hear those who killed her family calling out her name and searching the house to find her. But fortunately, they never did. Some time after the genocide, Immaculee visited the prison in her hometown where she asked to meet the man who had murdered her mother and brother. It was common practice for victims to come in and vent their anger and hatred against those who had committed such horrific crimes towards their loved ones. However, upon seeing him, Immaculee simply took his hands and told him she forgave him. When asked why, she said, 'Forgiveness is all I have to offer.' [21]

Ways to Be Compassionate

Research shows it's possible to learn how to be compassionate, and when you do, you are also more likely to be more accepting of yourself and others.

• **Practise Self-Compassion**

If you want to experience more compassion in your life or to be more compassionate towards others, the first step is to practise self-compassion – to notice when you are suffering, being critical of yourself, or treating yourself badly. And instead of ignoring what's happening or getting lost in a vacuum of self-pity, commit to being kind and loving towards yourself.

Experiencing emotional ups and downs, life's challenges, making mistakes, and not always getting the results you want, are all part of being human. None of us is perfect. In that moment, you always do the best you can, based on your emotional, mental, physical, spiritual health, and the resources available to you. You can't control all of what happens to you, but – if you choose to – you can make yourself feel better.

Examples of being compassionate to yourself include having a good work/ life balance; letting go of stresses, worries or anxieties; doing something that is healthy and makes you feel good (e.g. practising mindfulness or meditation; going for a walk, dancing, participating in sport); eating and drinking substances that nourish your body and spirit; getting creative (e.g. painting, singing, making something); reading or listening to music. In business, this could be charging good market prices for your services so you can earn a good living. Or you could do a job you enjoy.

• **Compassion Meditation**

Studies show that the regular practice of compassion meditation helps to reduce the levels of the stress hormone cortisol in the body. To do this, simply find somewhere quiet where you won't be disturbed, then get comfortable and close your eyes.

1. Become mindful and focus on your breathing, doing nothing other than letting your attention rest on how you are breathing for a few breaths.

---

21 *Left To Tell, Immaculee Ilibagiza, Hay House, 2006, p204.*

2. As you continue breathing, imagine feeling love in your heart.

3. Then imagine saying to every cell in your body, 'I love you… I wish you well… I'm here for you…'

4. Imagine thinking of people you love and saying to them, 'I love you… I wish you well… I'm here for you…'

5. When you're ready to do so, imagine people who have hurt you and say to them, 'I love you… I wish you well… I'm here for you…'

- **Perspectives Reflection**

Before responding or interacting with others, simply taking the time to reflect and acknowledge how they may be feeling can significantly transform the results you get, and help to avoid potential conflict.

We're all programmed with emotional triggers that automatically release undesirable responses when faced with challenging situations or behaviours. So the next time you are faced with a challenging event that would usually result in a negative reaction from you, before you respond take a few moments to consider:

- **What could they be scared of?**

- **What could they be troubled about?**

- **What pain or suffering could be triggering what they are doing?**

- **How could you respond in a way that demonstrates compassion?**

Compassion is closely linked to the heart values of love, kindness, respect, and peace, so practising the techniques I mentioned in these chapters too will certainly help build your capacity to feel and demonstrate compassion. In particular, I recommend using the exercise I mentioned in the last chapter, where you simply imagine feeling love, kindness, and compassion in your heart and then imagine 'sending' it to those who could benefit from it or who challenge you.

If you're in a relationship, you could complete this online Compassionate Love Quiz designed by The Greater Good Science Center at University of California, Berkley: http://greatergood.berkeley.edu/quizzes/take_quiz/9

Resourceful Questions

You may already be naturally compassionate in your approach to yourself and others, however it is worth taking a moment to consider the extent of this and to come up with more ideas. Be really honest and ask yourself the following questions:

- How am I compassionate towards myself?

- How could I be more compassionate towards myself?

- How could I be more compassionate towards others?

- Who do I find it hard to forgive?

- Who do I need to become to be more compassionate?

- To what extent do I feel hatred, anger or annoyance towards someone?

- How often am I fully present in the moment to recognise <u>and act upon</u> how others are feeling?

I know in the past I've seen appeals for help on TV when I've been in the middle of doing something else. I've felt the compassion in my heart and intended to make a donation, but not got round to it as I've been distracted by life around me. I hate it when I remember later that I forgot to call and make a donation. However, having that awareness has triggered a change in my behaviour, so now, if possible, I stop what I am doing at the time and make a donation immediately.

How could you be more compassionate in the moment?

Empowering Affirmations To Nurture Your Heart

- I release the past and forgive everyone.

- I naturally feel compassion in my heart.

- I'm getting better each day at treating myself with compassion.

- I feel good when I take action to eliminate others' suffering.

- I am compassionate towards those who challenge or hurt me.

Tapping 'Set Up' Statements

- Even though I sometimes don't notice how others are feeling, I deeply and completely accept myself.

- Even though I sometimes don't know what to do to help others, I deeply and completely accept myself.

- Even though I feel no-one cares about what I'm going through, I know I can learn to feel better about myself, and the situation I'm in.

Recommended Resources

- *The Compassionate Mind* by Paul Gilbert
- *The Dalai Lama's Book Of Wisdom* edited by Matthew E. Bunson
- *The Divine Matrix* by Gregg Braden
- *Left To Tell* by Immaculee Ilibagiza
- The Charter For Compassion - http://charterforcompassion.org/
- *Nonviolent Communication, A Language Of Life* by Marshall B. Rosenberg PHD

Chapter 8

Principle 1 – Heart Value – Integrity

Be true and authentic to the pure essence of who you were born to be.

Are you being true to yourself in all areas of your life? Or are you are compromising your truth in any way?

Every week I speak to people who are unhappy about something they are tolerating in their life:

• a job they don't like

• a relationship that no longer brings them joy

• avoiding doing what they know needs to be done

• feeling 'disconnected' to the person they used to be or know is within them

• others' negative behaviour towards them

• their own unhappiness or poor health

You were born into this world with endless possibilities and the potential to be a wonderful unique being. But from that day on, other people have shaped and moulded you into someone who fits into family, community, and cultural expectations – affecting what you think, what you do, what you say, how you feel, what you wear, what you value, etc. And unless you've proactively taken action to re-align your life to the true essence of who you are, the likelihood is that you've become detached from this to some extent.

Living a life of integrity is about speaking your truth – through your actions and your words. And at a deeper level, it's about re-connecting to your soul so that your words and actions are aligned to your highest truth and interests – your pure authentic self.

When I think back to the time when I worked in the investment industry, I'm amazed I was able to last in that arena for so long. Not only did I have a huge values clash with many colleagues who were driven mainly by status, money, or what this could buy, when I'm not. But I also allowed myself to dress, talk, and act in a way that was not a true reflection of me. In order to fit into what felt like an alien world, I compromised what was important to me, what I loved to do, what energised me, and what fed my soul. To the extent that after fifteen years I no longer 'knew' who I was. I just felt as though my life had no meaning. And so I jumped at the chance of redundancy so I could explore and reconnect to the lost soul inside me, and to make changes in my life that would create a lifestyle reflecting the true essence of who I am. One of the first things I did was to give all my 'corporate land' suits to a charity shop and replace them with colourful clothes that better reflected my true personality. I still sometimes do training consultancy in this industry, but now have the confidence to be myself and only work with those who share similar values.

Do you know who your true authentic self is?

When you are living a life of integrity, you say what you think, you express what you feel, and you take action that is completely aligned to this. You do not tolerate things in your life because you are scared of the potential consequences of taking action (e.g. being alone, not having enough money, the uncertainty it could bring, what people may think or do). Being 'out of' integrity means holding back on expressing what you really think; saying one thing but doing something that conflicts with this; putting your head in the sand; saying what you think others want to hear, rather than what you'd really like to say; and avoiding doing what you know needs to be done.

'Have the courage to say no. Have the courage to face the truth. Do the right thing because it is right. These are the magic keys to living your life with integrity.'

W Clement Stone, Businessman & Author

Investing too much time and energy helping or caring for others, or doing what we think is expected of us at a cost to our own health, happiness, and wellbeing, can result in feelings of resentment, unhappiness, depression, worthiness, and a lack of interest in life. Often this can happen unintentionally when we jump wholeheartedly into roles such as parent, partner, spouse or employee, and give up a part of ourselves to fulfil these roles. If you're choosing to take on certain roles, e.g. having children or caring for a loved one (and all that entails) because doing so is really important to you, then that is in alignment with your values and truth – as long as you balance this with being honest in every moment of these and remember to connect with the essence of who you are, too. Because the more you remain true to yourself when taking on these responsibilities, the happier, healthier, and more capable you'll be.

How to Be More Aligned to Your Truth

The first step of aligning to your truth is to identify the areas where you're not being true to yourself, and taking action to re-align your integrity. The scale of action required depends on how much you've been compromising who you are and what's important to you.

So start by asking yourself:

- In what way(s) am I not being true to myself?

- In what way(s) am I not being true to others?

- What am I avoiding?

- What am I tolerating?

- What have I said I'll do that I haven't done yet?

- What's important to me?

- Who do I love being?

- What do I love doing?

Once you've identified how you're not aligned to your truth, you can take action to remedy this. Examples of how you can do this include:

- having conversations you've been avoiding

- doing what you said you would do but have not yet done

- speaking up if you don't agree with what someone else has said

- taking the time to rediscover what you love to do and your life purpose – Chapter 13

- making the time to do what's important to you

- leaving an abusive relationship (personal, or in the workplace)

- tackling whatever you've been tolerating (e.g. behaviours, relationships, unfinished business/tasks, mess).

Taking this to the next level, once you know who you are (your beliefs, what's important to you, what you love, and how you want to make an impact in the world), it's much easier to voice your opinions and take appropriate action. But this is obviously only possible once you've also developed the self-belief and conviction that who you are inside IS important. That you are a unique and special being who deserves to be heard, loved, treated well, feel happy, and be successful. And you are already – right now!

You will learn ways to rediscover and reconnect to your natural and authentic self in Chapters 12 and 13.

Resourceful Questions

Be really honest and ask yourself the following questions to give you ideas how to be more authentic:

- How could I be more true to myself?

- How could I be more honest with others?

- In what way am I not living a life of integrity?

- In what way am I not being completely true to others?

- What could I do to be acting more in line with my values?

Empowering Affirmations to Nurture Your Heart

- I deserve to be happy and successful being me!

- I love feeling truly connected to my authentic self.

- I say what I think, with kindness and compassion.

- I let someone know if I don't agree with what they've said or done.

- I always do what I say I'll do.

Tapping 'Set Up' Statements

- Even though I find it hard to say what I really think, I deeply and completely accept I always do the best I can.

- Even though I sometimes don't feel good enough, I deeply and completely love and accept myself.

- Even though I sometimes avoid what I know I need to do, I deeply and completely love and accept myself.

Chapter 9

Principle 1 – Heart Value – Respect

Treat yourself with respect, be mindful of and honour others' rights and opinions

I love spending time having fun and chatting with my friends about all sorts of things. And because we have such a diverse range of interests, it's not surprising that differing points of view sometimes arise. I remember first noticing this – as a teenager – with someone who is still one of my dearest friends. We used to have very different tastes in fashion that often meant if she liked something, I didn't, and vice versa. Thankfully, we found a way of having fun while being honest with one another, in a heartfelt way. One of the reasons I cherish our friendship is that, despite very different life experiences and interests as adults, I have a deep love, affinity, and respect for her. We both feel comfortable saying what we think, and value what each other has to say, because we know it is coming from a place of love and wanting the best for each other. I'm so grateful to her for being such a special friend in my life. Because, as I'm sure you'll have experienced, not all relationships are this way.

Have you ever held back from saying what you think because you've been concerned about what others could think? Or have you realised that you've acted in a way that wasn't the kindest response to how others were feeling?

Someone who has self-respect takes responsibility for nurturing their mind, body, and soul; for treating themselves in a way they'd like others to treat them; for living a life of integrity; for having high personal standards that they live up to; and for setting healthy personal boundaries relating to how they allow others to treat them.

In their interactions with others, they seek to listen to and value others' opinions (even if different to their own) and to treat others in a way that's at least as good as they'd like to be treated themselves. They see beyond titles, roles, status, perceived wealth, actions, and behaviours, and accept everyone as the soul of potential they are inside. An extension of this is to treat all living creatures and the planet in this way too – to have a respect for all aspects of life.

> *'Treat people with dignity and respect, even if you don't know them and even if you don't agree with them.'*
>
> ### Michelle Obama

As we've all had different life experiences, it's natural that we all have differing views and opinions. But who's to say which is right or wrong? Countries today have plenty of cultural values that differ from views of only a few decades ago, and which are different from many other countries. Even within each country there are a diverse range of opinions and thoughts about almost every topic.

As I write this chapter, the 2014 Winter Olympics in Sochi, Russia, have just started amid global controversy relating the attitudes of many of Russia's leaders towards the gay community. Many of their comments, actions, and behaviours do not appear to respect human rights and are instead cultivating discriminatory violence in their country, similar to that committed by the Nazis ahead of World War II. While this appalls many of us who live in societies that equally value all human life irrespective of sexual orientation, it's worth remembering that those who believe otherwise have been conditioned to think differently through their life experiences. Unfortunately it takes time to influence a change in cultural beliefs, with respectful dialogue and education programmes.

Your perspective is simply based upon your own life experiences, the associations you've developed, and cultural 'norms' you've chosen to adopt – whether at a family, community, workplace or national level. This is a unique blend of what you've learned to think, feel, and believe to be true. However, because we're all running a different life movie in our minds, we will always have different ways to think and feel about every situation. If you want to enjoy more fulfilling long-term relationships and success, it's important to be mindful of how you respond when variances arise.

The more open-minded you are in respecting others' perspectives and their right to be treated with love, compassion and respect, the greater the likelihood that your own relationships and life will be harmonious – particularly when you have a healthy balance between self-respect and respecting others – when you accept each and every person as a unique and wonderful being, irrespective of nationality, religious beliefs, social status, gender, education, age, sexual preference, physical ability, and any other way you categorise people.

When people are being respectful to you, you are likely to feel:

• free to express what you truly think and feel

• you are being treated in a way you like to be treated

• you are being listened to and that your point of view has been heard

• that what you need and want is being taken into account

• you have a choice

• you are being treated with kindness and compassion.

By contrast, those who choose to adopt a narrow-minded approach and believe that their way of thinking is the only 'right' way, are more likely to experience more problems, disagreements, challenges, conflict, unhappiness, and frustration in life. They may:

• talk 'over' you or 'at' you, with no interest in what you're thinking or feeling

• react negatively when you say 'no' nicely to them (about something it is perfectly reasonable for you to say 'no' to)

• be aggressive, hostile, or humiliate you

• demand your respect while being disrespectful to you

• make you feel you 'have to' or 'should' do something that you don't want to do

• turn up uninvited, and expect or demand that you stop what you're doing.

I remember once at work, a young member of my team asked whether he needed to respect a colleague who was older than him but whose behaviours he found offensive. He had been taught to respect his elders as a default, while others (of a similar or younger age or social standing) needed to earn his respect. However, he was being challenged because a more senior manager was not treating him and other colleagues well, often demonstrating what others perceived as aggressive and insulting behaviour. The young man was finding it hard to respect someone with very different values and who was demonstrating a lack of respect towards him.

This highlights the distinction between respecting others and being respectful. It is natural in life to encounter people you may dislike and find hard to respect, particularly if they have views or act in a way that clashes with your values and what you consider to be acceptable. In situations when you don't agree with others' perspective or actions, sometimes the only thing to respect is that they are a living human being with the right to live, and let this form the foundation for a respectful response.

Often in Rwanda when we are making our way up the dirt track road from the capital Kigali to a remote orphanage on a mountaintop outside, we pass many of those who were culpable during the genocide. As part of their restitution, they have been tasked with upgrading the road. It's hard manual work, often in heavy monsoon rain or the blistering heat of the sun. When we pass these thin, aged men, the overseas contingent of our team acknowledge, smile, and wave to them. And it's lovely to see flickers of joy on some of their faces for being greeted with compassion, because they are so used to being ignored by most Rwandans, many of whom find it hard to show compassion or respect towards them.

Now let's be clear – I have absolutely no idea how I'd feel and cope if I came face-to-face with anyone responsible for killing members of my family or friends. But I do know, from working with others, that one of the most powerful ways to heal our emotional wounds is to open our hearts; come from a place of kindness and compassion; and be open to the possibility that people who commit such acts, must themselves have been through terrible suffering. I really do try to avoid judging others, especially when I have no idea how I'd act to protect myself or loved ones if under threat.

Do I respect people who commit such crimes? Of course I don't respect their actions, but I aim to respect the pure essence at the core of every human being, and to be respectful in my interaction with them. Being respectful isn't about 'liking' or respecting everything about the other person. It's about choosing to interact with peace, compassion, and respect towards those you encounter. It means respecting their human rights, irrespective of their attitudes, actions, and behaviours. And balancing this with the need for self-defence, obviously!

How would it be if you could respect everyone as a default, for the purest essence, life source, and potential within? That even if you didn't respect them as a person, their actions or behaviour, you could act with kindness, compassion, and be respectful towards them?

Activating all the other heart values is a way to nurture an attitude of respect – in that, if you come from a place of love, kindness, compassion, integrity, and peace when interacting with others, you're likely to be respectful.

An indicator of how much you respect yourself versus others, is your propensity to be assertive. Professor and author Maureen Guirdham defines assertive as 'standing up for our own rights in such a way that you do not violate another person's rights'.

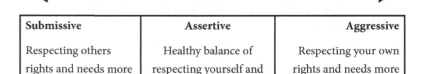

Submissive	Assertive	Aggressive
Respecting others rights and needs more than your own	Healthy balance of respecting yourself and others	Respecting your own rights and needs more than others

When you are assertive, you are operating from a healthy balance of respecting yourself and others, so you are likely to feel good, have happier relationships, and to get results without hurting others. However, it often takes courage to be honest and say or do what will bring you equilibrium, because of the potential consequences of doing so.

Those who respect others more than themselves often let others violate their rights and take advantage of them, e.g. do what they are told to do (rather than deciding what to do themselves or collaboratively); go along with others' plans at the sacrifice of their own goals; or allow others to shout, hurt or be unkind to them. Benefits of being submissive include avoiding conflict, uncertainty, and the need to take responsibility. But regularly choosing to be submissive can lead to feelings of frustration, hurt, anger, upset, resentment, worthlessness, doubt, anxiety, and other negative emotions. You may also feel dis-satisfied with your life and experience unfulfilling relationships.

If you ever express aggression towards others, in those moments you are violating their rights – in other words, you are not respecting their thoughts, feelings or needs. You may get things done in the short-term, but you could be achieving your goals at the expense of others, and be someone others don't want to be around longer term.

You may be assertive in some situations yet submissive or aggressive in others. And, of course, demonstrating respect towards others isn't always about being assertive.

Have you ever got to the checkout of your local supermarket and found there are people at the end of the counter who are collecting money on behalf of a charity or social club? While I'm a great fan of youngsters contributing to their cause and raising money for charity, I don't feel it's respectful to shoppers to have bag-packers on every checkout – especially for people who are counting their pennies, may not have the extra money for this, and yet feel social pressure to make a donation.

In this situation, having two young people standing at the end of a checkout would rarely be described as being aggressive, but to some extent it takes away an element of choice. I understand that as a fundraising strategy, it clearly works better than having a bucket which people walk past. However, I wonder if it's more respectful to offer people a choice by having some without packers too. Intentionally putting pressure on people for any reason doesn't feel right to me.

You are more likely to enjoy success when you balance respect for yourself with respect for others. Aggressive or submissive behaviours are more likely to sabotage your long-term chances of happiness and success.

How to Respect Yourself and Be Assertive

1. **Set personal standards** – take time to decide how you will treat yourself, to put yourself in the best place for success and living a happy, healthy and meaningful life. This could include deciding what to eat and drink; how to keep yourself fit; how you interact with others; knowing what's important to you; standing up for yourself (respectfully); and overcoming self-doubt and criticism.

2. **Set boundaries** – decide how you'd like others to treat you, in terms of acceptable and unacceptable behaviours. For example, the following would be unacceptable behaviours to me – shouting at me, physically hurting me, lying to me, ignoring what I'm saying, not valuing my opinions, embarrassing me in front of others, or putting me down.

3. **Speak up** – when you have an opinion to share, whenever someone is being disrespectful to you, or to reduce the potential for conflict where there are differing opinions. The UHT model is a really useful tool to help work out what you say to others:

- **U = Understand (alternative words could be realise, sense, hear, see, feel, know)**

- **H = However (or but)**

- **T = Therefore**

Examples of how to use this include:

- **I understand that you'd like me to come and see you on Saturday, however I've got something else on I've already arranged. Therefore, how about I come round on Sunday evening instead?**

- **I realise you'd like me to XXX, but I don't like the way you're talking to me. Therefore, let's talk about this when you've calmed down.**

- **I realise you think XXX is the best way forward, but I think YYY would work better. How about we arrange a meeting or time to discuss this further?**

A Few Tips For Respecting Others:

- Treat others in a way that is at least as good as you'd like them to treat you – irrespective of how they are treating you (unless of course your life is in danger, in which case you need to do whatever you can to save your life).

- Do what you can to put yourself in a positive emotional 'state' (e.g. one of love, kindness or compassion) ahead of interactions with others. Particularly with 'difficult' or challenging people.

- Ask others what they think and feel (and respect this), rather than speaking 'at' them or forcing yourself upon them.

- Where you have a difference of opinion, you could say, 'I respect that you think/feel XXX, therefore how about we agree to disagree?'

Resourceful Questions

Be really honest and ask yourself the following questions to give you ideas how you could be more respectful:

- How could you be more respectful towards yourself?

- Are there any people you are submissive around?

- Are there are any people you are aggressive towards?

- How could you be more assertive?

- How could you be more respectful towards others?

- When do you express anger or frustration?

Empowering Affirmations to Nurture Your Heart

- I love and respect myself the way I am.

- I speak up with confidence when I have something to say.

- I let others know if I am unhappy with something they have said or done.

- I treat myself in a way that I'd love others to treat me.

Tapping 'Set Up' Statements

- Even though I'm sometimes scared to speak up, I deeply and completely accept I always do the best I can.

- Even though I sometimes act in a way I later regret, I deeply and completely love and accept myself.

- Even though I put others' needs before mine too much, I realise I can change this.

Recommended Resources

- *Nonviolent Communication, A Language Of Life* by Marshall B. Rosenberg PHD

Chapter 10

Principle 1 – Heart Value – Gratitude

Be appreciative and express gratitude

Every day, I count my blessings with deep appreciation in my heart. Not just on the days when life is going really well but even more so on the days when it's not. Why? Because I've learned that gratitude and appreciation are wonderful remedies for feeling down, scared, or finding it hard to cope with life's challenges. That when life gets difficult, I have a choice – to wallow in self-pity, complain, or blame others for what's happening. Or to pick myself up and focus on what I am grateful for.

I remember using the practice of gratitude as a natural pick-me-up strategy during my divorce. I was determined that while I was terribly sad that my first marriage hadn't worked out as I'd dreamt it would, I didn't want to feel bad any longer than I had to. A particularly challenging day was a few days after my ex-husband moved out and I was to deliver a 'Pure Happiness' Workshop at one of my client's offices. As a professional trainer, I wanted to ensure the participants experienced the usual fun, uplifting, and transformational day – yet inside I was feeling sick to the core. I knew I had to change my emotional state for the day, so on the way through to Glasgow on the train I sat and wrote a list of all the things I was grateful for in my life – I was alive, I was healthy, I had a way of earning income and could support myself, I had a great circle of friends who were rallying around, I had my family's support, my family were all healthy, and that I knew I'd done the best I could to make my marriage work.

Included in this list were the many things I was grateful for relating to my marriage – the many happy times we'd had together, for the friends I'd met through my ex-husband, and for the love and affection I still felt for him. Yes, I was still sad and upset, but as I focused on what I was grateful for, I noticed the harshness of my sadness began to lessen. Taking the time to contemplate all I was grateful for helped me feel better in the moment so that I could carry on the day with more positive energy. And I had to laugh to myself later that day when over lunch one of the group asked, 'Is there is ever a day when you don't feel happy and what you're teaching doesn't work?'

I think of gratitude in two ways – the first being to emotionally feel thanks or appreciation in your heart, and the second being to outwardly express thanks to others. Internally, it's a celebration of the present moment that you feel naturally or can consciously choose to feel (particularly at times when you'd like to feel better about a situation that's churning up negative emotions).

Studies show that putting yourself into an emotional state of gratitude or appreciation can help prevent illness, boost your immune system, aid the healing process, and boost your emotional wellbeing (including happiness and optimism). That's because when you feel grateful, your body produces hormones that do you good, such as endorphins and oxytocin, rather than hormones such as adrenalin, cortisol, and norepinephrine that are damaging to your health over the long-term.

And according to author Dr David Hamilton, you're more likely to achieve personal goals because 'we feel more motivated when we feel good but we are also more creative and more likely to spot solutions to our problems'.[22] And so being able to be in a state of gratitude whenever you choose to be, not only feels good in the moment, but it also has lots of other health benefits.

Being appreciative often also results in us being more thoughtful, forgiving, and generous in our actions towards others. By contemplating the good in a person or situation, you shift your focus and this will help you see things from a different perspective and feel better. This in turn can help you overcome negative emotions (such as depression, fear, anger, worry or resentment) so you can be more effective in the moment.

As I write this chapter, I've been practicing gratitude for asbestos.

22 Dr David Hamilton Blog, 10 Reasons Why Gratitude Is Good For You, January 2014, www.drdavidhamilton.com

My husband and I have always talked about retiring to a gorgeous Scottish village by the sea, and the opportunity came up to buy our ideal house there a few years early. As you can imagine, we were really excited to get the keys. But within only ten minutes of starting the refurbishment, one young lad from the building company discovered what he thought was asbestos – and he was right. It transpired that our house was held up by asbestos joists. Over the next three weeks, we encountered problem after problem. To the extent that we decided to strip out most of the floors, ceilings, and walls inside, in order to create an asbestos-free home. Currently we have an outer shell and a staircase to nowhere!

It has been a challenging time as I've stepped into project managing the rebuild a couple of days a week and re-jigging our plans around fast dwindling savings. But it wasn't until my mum commented about how resilient we were being that I realised, yes we have been. Partly because of the support we have around us, but also because I now automatically use many of the tools I'm sharing with you in this book. And from the minute it was confirmed we had asbestos, one of the things I did was to list all the things I was grateful for about the situation – that being self-employed I have the flexibility to create the time to oversee what's happening; that we're not ripping out anything new (which would have happened if we'd discovered it further down the line); that while we may not get our extension built this year, we will be able to create a lovely home in a great location; that I can escape to the beach within a few minutes; that it's made me focus better on cash generating activities in my business; that I'm working fewer hours; that I'm using my brain differently (and enjoying that). And most importantly, to have the perspective that while it's an expensive hassle we'd prefer to have done without, it is at least something that can get sorted out, unlike some other life challenges.

I'm also grateful to have learned how powerful gratitude can be in this respect – to have fairly quickly moved through feeling upset and worried, to one of acceptance then gratitude. The 'old me' (the younger version of myself who didn't know this was a strategy I could use for this type of situation) would have spent weeks worried and stressed about what was happening, not sleeping, and wondering 'why me?'. But that would only have had a negative impact on my own emotional and physical health (I would probably have been opening more bottles of wine, too), and would have wasted time and energy doing things that would have slowed down progress.

And over the longer-term, research even shows that gratitude can help prevent such negative emotions and increase your emotional resilience when faced with challenging life events.[23] Or as Anthony Robins once said, 'When you are grateful, fear disappears and abundance appears.'

So choosing to feel gratitude can be used as a strategy to change how you feel and to help you become more consciously aware of your thoughts, the impact that they have, and to put what you're experiencing into perspective with what's really important.

Practicing gratitude and appreciation is also about taking the time to express thanks to others. How often do you take the time to share your appreciation for something or say 'thank-you' with a comment, card, or letter?

'Feeling gratitude and not expressing it is like wrapping a present and not giving it.'

William Arthur Ward, American Author

I'm frequently surprised at how ungrateful people can be towards others, and especially those who are helping them out.

For example, when I get off a bus, I always thank the driver who has helped me reach my destination, but I notice that many people don't. A lot of the time people may not set out to ignore the driver, but rather they are disconnected to the present moment (e.g. because they are distracted by their thoughts, or using mobile devices) and just don't think.

How often do you say thanks?

How often do others thank you?

Most people don't hear enough praise nor are thanked enough.

So I encourage you to consciously look up, enjoy the present moment, and connect with others – saying hello, being kind, or expressing your gratitude. Taking the time to say thanks, sending a card, letter or email, is such a simple thing for you to do but could make a huge difference, not just to you but also to others.

And if you're in a position where you have influence on how others feel, e.g.

23 Robert Emmons, *Professor Psychology US Davis, What Good Is Gratitude?, Greater Good Science Center, YouTube Channel*

as a parent, teacher, leader, manager, consider how you could use gratitude to help them feel good:

I remember discussing gratitude with a group of teachers and being really encouraged by what one of them did with her class of 7-8-year-olds. She told us how one of the hardest things about her job was not being able to do as much as she'd like to do for the children who appeared to experience neglect, lack of love or kindness, and possibly worse, at home. She knew all she could do was give the children the best experience she could during the day, and she resolved to do whatever she could to have them leave feeling good at the end of the day. And one of the things she got her class to do each afternoon was to write down and share what they were grateful for that day. Whilst she never knew how much of a difference doing this made, the children in her class seemed to really enjoy doing this and she felt she'd done the best she could.

Ways to Feel Grateful

1. Personal Gratitude Reflection

Whenever you feel challenged, take a moment to reflect and consider what you are grateful for about the situation. You may also want to write this down – especially if it's about something more challenging, or that you need to deal with on an on-going basis.

If you are particularly upset or feeling another strong negative emotion, you may first wish to do some tapping (see Chapter 22) to put yourself in a better emotional state more quickly, before writing down what you're grateful for.

Tapping and practicing gratitude are now usually the first two strategies that I use to help me let go of stress and cope better with challenging situations/people.

2. Gratitude Journal

Regularly write down a list of all the things you're feeling grateful for in a special notebook for this purpose, or in your Success Journal. To do this, simply write 'I'm so grateful for...' at the top of the page, and see what comes into your mind. Write down whatever comes up.

Sometimes it can be difficult to come up with things to be grateful for when we have been really hurt or are very upset, so a starting point may be to list the generic basics of life, e.g. I am alive, I have food and water, I have a roof over my head, etc. By doing this, you'll open your mind to the possibility of gratitude, and once you get going you may find it easier to come up with other things to be grateful for.

There are several ways to practise gratitude, and several studies have been carried out into the effectiveness of writing a gratitude journal. What's important is that you work out what works for you:

- Some people like to do this at the end of a day – taking a few minutes to reflect and be grateful for that day's events can put you in a better frame of mind before drifting off to sleep than watching a horror movie or the news.

  However, some studies report that contemplating what you're grateful for each day reduces the effectiveness of this practice over time, because we adapt to the positive feelings that we've previously noted down.

  You may find that writing in detail about a particular thing, person or event you're grateful for is more effective than writing a large superficial list.

- Noting down what you're grateful for that *didn't* happen may also help you feel a deeper sense of appreciation for a situation, as could noting down the benefits that have come from what could otherwise be perceived as a challenging or 'bad' situation.

Ways to Express Gratitude

A bit like practicing kindness, expressing gratitude may be something that you already do. However, you may want to consider whether there are ways you can:

- say thanks more often

- express thanks in a way that will be best received by the other person (e.g. in their love language that I referred to in Chapter 5)

- surprise someone with a card, letter or email

Resourceful Questions

Be really honest and ask yourself the following questions about how you could be more appreciative in life.

- What am I grateful for (and why)?

- Who am I grateful to (and why)?

- When could I show more appreciation?

- What are the positive outcomes of this challenging situation?

- Who could I say thank you to today?

Empowering Affirmations to Nurture Your Heart

- I am so grateful for…

- I love spending time updating my gratitude journal.

- I treat all challenging situations/people as opportunities for growth.

- I'm blessed…

- I really appreciate the support I have from those around me.

Tapping 'Set Up' Statements

- Even though I can't find anything good about XXX, I deeply and completely accept myself.

- Even though I'm not feeling grateful right now, I know I can change how I feel.

- Even though I'm really upset about XXX, I am glad to be alive.

Recommended Resources

- *Why Kindness Is Good For You* by Dr David R Hamilton

- The Greater Good Science Center – http://greatergood.berkeley.edu/

Download Your Free Gratitude Relaxation Audio

If you'd like to let go of stress or feel good for a few moments, my gift to you is a short relaxation exercise that you can download for free from my website. Go to http://www.alisoun.com/heartatude to find out more.

Chapter 11

Principle 1 – Heart Value – Peace

Release the past, be forgiving, and let go of future worries.

If you want to experience peace in any area of your life, mastering how to feel it in your heart and how to act in a way that reflects this, will help you enjoy more peace. This can include enjoying more harmonious relationships and living or working in a peaceful environment.

'One day we must come to see that peace is not merely a distant goal we seek, but that it is a means by which we arrive at that goal. We must pursue peaceful ends through peaceful means.' [24]

Martin Luther King Jr., Human Rights Activist & Noble Prize Winner

When you choose to believe that every one of us always does the best we can, in every moment, based upon the resources available to us at that time, you develop a new sense of peace in your heart. Combine this with letting go of doubts, worries, fears, anxieties, guilt, and other negative thoughts and feelings, about the past, present and future, and you'll feel more content and at peace with yourself, towards others, and in many situations in your life. Those around you are also more likely to react positively to you because they'll be picking up and reflecting your calm and positive personal energy.

What you feel about the past and future is triggered by all your thoughts, memories, and associations about everything you've experienced since the day you were born. Neutralising any negative emotional charges will enable you to feel inner peace in your heart.

24 *http://mlk-kpp01.stanford.edu/index.php/resources/article/king_quotes_on_war_and_peace/*

Peace in this context is about letting go of thoughts and emotions about the past and future, so you can be fully present in the moment and choose to act from a place of pure love, kindness, and compassion in your heart. When you master this, you'll notice you feel calmer in response to what's happening around you.

Frequently, you may not be aware of what is triggering your feelings, actions and behaviours, because these are driven by what's stored in your mind at an unconscious level. However, your body will let you know whether or not you're living from a place of peace in your heart. The following behaviours indicate when it could be beneficial for you to heal wounds from the past:

• being critical of yourself

• being critical towards others

• shouting, being violent, or attacking others

• experiencing feelings of doubt, stress, anxiety, fear, anger, frustration, resentment, hurt, judgment, hatred, guilt, disappointment, or regret

• finding it hard to move on from the past, or to be able to forgive someone.

So, feeling peace in the present moment is about letting go of negative thoughts and emotions relating to the past and future. Choosing to come from a place of love, kindness and compassion will help you do this, and you'll find out more about how to manage your thoughts and feelings in Chapter 15. A starting point is to become more mindful of how you are every day – to pay attention to the clues you get from what you are doing or feeling.

In terms of success, have you ever given in to personal doubt and, as a result, not achieved a goal or outcome you really wanted? Would it have been more beneficial to let go of these thoughts, and instead taken resourceful action more aligned to your goal?

If there is an area of your life where you're not happy, I encourage you to learn how to manage your emotions and to find peace in your heart – towards yourself and others. That's not to say this is easy. Often it isn't, particularly if that involves finding the strength within you to be more courageous or to embark upon an emotional journey of self-healing. That is where the art of acceptance and forgiveness is one of the most empowering perspectives you can master in life.

'When you forgive, it doesn't mean that you condone what people are doing wrong, but you can still forgive them, let go the anger, let go the bitterness and accept to have your peace.'

Immaculee Illibaguza, Author & Genocide Survivor

I remember the first time someone suggested forgiving people I felt had 'done me an injustice'. I couldn't understand why I would ever want to do this. At that time, it felt as though forgiving them would be communicating to them that they were 'right' to have done what they did.

However, I have since learned that forgiveness is nothing to do with condoning what someone else has done – it's about releasing yourself so that you are free to move forward with your life, with love in your heart. Holding onto resentment, anger, and bitterness is a sure way to extend your hurt and pain when you don't need to. Such feelings sabotage your chances of being truly happy, and can seriously damage your health. However, opening your heart to feelings such as peace, love, kindness and compassion, will elevate how you feel and raise your energy vibration for success.

Part of being human is that sometimes we do make mistakes, or do things we wish we'd done differently. In those situations, it's how you choose to interpret those experiences which has an impact on how you feel. Are you prone to feeling regret, disappointment or guilt? Or do you choose to accept you did the best you could, based upon the resources you had available at the time (skills, energy, tools, strength, money, time, experience, perspective, etc.)?

'The practice of forgiveness is our most important contribution to the healing of the world.' [25]

Marianne Williamson, Spiritual Teacher

What I love about the work we do in Rwanda is that by helping to heal the wounds of war, we are creating a ripple in the quest for world peace. By learning to 'forgive', the young people we work with have found love and peace in their hearts again and are more likely to enjoy living in peace. By contrast, many not letting go of hatred, anger or resentment in extreme cases is what fuels violence, terrorism and starts wars.

Sometimes being at peace is also accepting that there are some things you can't control in your life.

---

[25] http://www.goodreads.com/quotes/119843-the-practice-of-forgiveness-is-our-most-important-contribution-to

A few weeks ago I had a reiki session with a special friend who, as usual at the start, asked how I was. I explained that I'd been trying to work out what drove me to work the long hours I'd been doing (other than my love for my work). After a pause, her response was 'forgiveness', and she suggested that I contemplate who and what I needed to forgive during my treatment. Knowing from experience that her intuition is often right, I did just that, and was stunned by what came up – that I needed to forgive myself for not having had children. In the previous years, I'd chosen to fill this void with other activities – including my humanitarian work and holidays – and thought I'd accepted it. But what I discovered that day was that I still 'blamed' my inability to have children on not being a good enough person to be a mum, that most others manage it so therefore there had to be something wrong with me (when medically, no reason was found to be a contributing factor). Now I'd never consciously thought that I wasn't a good enough person to have children, but for whatever reason it had been bubbling away in my unconscious mind. And that's where I am so grateful to know many ways to tackle the issues or blocks that are hindering my success – the techniques I'm sharing with you in this book. In this case, I chose to do a couple of NLP techniques and some tapping on myself, to forgive myself for having such thoughts. By being curious and taking remedial action, I've since felt a lot more grounded, calm, and balanced in my approach to my work.

How to Enjoy More Peace in Your Life

In Rwanda, we teach many of the heart values I'm sharing with you in this book – particularly those of love, compassion and forgiveness – using a number of approaches, including 'tapping' and 'The Grace Process' – developed by my great friend Dr Lori Leyden (founder of Create Global Healing, with whom I go to Rwanda). The Grace Process is based on five healing elements you can embrace every day, and which I share here with Lori's express permission:

1. **Intention** – choose to live in the beauty and wonder of what this life was meant to be, and create the most expansive intentions for manifesting the healing or miracle you desire.
2. **Releasing judgment** – become aware of any and all judgments you may have about yourself, others, and the circumstances in which you find yourself.
3. **Forgiveness** – forgive yourself, others, and the circumstances in which you find yourself.

4.   **Heart resonance** – hold within your heart the highest resonance of gratitude, love, joy and wonder, in as many moments as possible, as you co-create your intentions.

5.   **Receiving and harnessing grace** – receive and honour the miracle and gifts all around you as you live in the energy of Grace. Welcome the transformation of your healing and the realisation of your intentions.

I'm sure you'll have realised by now that the first step in experiencing more peace in your life is (as with the other Principles) to consider how you can change yourself – and particularly when you experience others' behaviours that don't reflect this approach.

Personally, I found that it was easier to start releasing the small feelings of regret, anger, and disappointment, etc, before tackling the bigger emotional issues. Depending on what you've experienced in life, finding peace in your heart could be an emotional journey. So, please do be kind to yourself! Do get the support of a professional therapist if you feel you need help in moving forward.

You may wish to start by using some of the following resourceful questions, affirmations, or tapping statements:

Resourceful Questions

Be honest and ask yourself the following questions to give you ideas how you could feel more inner peace:

• What do I feel bad about or regret?

• What bad experiences do I dwell on from the past?

• Who do I worry about?

• How could I be more forgiving towards others?

• How could I better accept we all do the best we can?

Empowering Affirmations to Nurture Your Heart

• I always do the best I can with the resources I have available at any point in time.

• I know others always do the best they can.

• I release the past and forgive everyone.

- I'm getting better at letting go of doubts, worries and anxieties every day.

- I'm so glad I know I can cope with whatever life throws at me.

Tapping 'Set-Up' Statements

- Even though I find it hard to forgive myself, I accept I do the best I can.

- Even though I worry about the future, I know I can learn to let this go.

- Even though I hold onto the past, I deeply and completely accept myself.

Recommended Resources

- *The Grace Process Guidebook* by Dr Lori Leyden PhD

- The EFT Personal Peace Procedure – see *The EFT Manual* by Gary Craig/ Dawson Church

Chapter 12

Principle 2 – Make A Difference

Align your actions to have a positive impact – for you, others, the world, and the planet. Stepping up to share your unique gifts, skills, and qualities in ways that you are of best support, service or value to your family, clients, colleagues, organisation, or whatever cause is important to you.

There's a lovely story about a man walking along a beach. He's taking in the fresh air, enjoying the views and listening to the soothing sounds of the waves breaking on the sand and rocks. As he glances up, he notices a woman in the distance, interrupting her walk every few steps by bending down, then standing up and throwing something into the sea. Initially the man wonders what she's doing, until he gets nearer and sees that the sand around her is scattered with starfish. As he approaches her, he stops and asks, 'What are you doing? There are hundreds of starfish stranded on the sand, you're never going to make much difference.' She smiles and, as she throws the next starfish into the sea, replies, 'But I can make a difference to that one.'

I am full of great respect and admiration for those who embrace 'giving back' to society and dedicate a significant part of their life to all sorts of causes, including those who adopt children; are doing good in local communities, humanitarian and voluntary work; men and women in the Forces; inventors and those working in labs seeking cures to many modern day diseases. All our lives are enriched by those who focus on making a difference to others.

But what does 'making a difference' have to do with success?

It's a strange world when those who make money for companies that have a negative impact on the world are paid high salaries, whilst those doing so much good are often expected to do it for nothing or for pennies. I hear many people expressing how they want the charitable donations they make to go directly to those who need it, and not those running or working in the charities. Why do so many expect those working for charitable causes to do it for nothing, when without them no-one would benefit? Not valuing their work and those who truly make a positive impact seems madness to me – are they not some of the people most deserving of good salaries?

There are many people who set themselves goals for what they'd like to achieve in their life – personally, or through their work. But, I've always felt a slight disconnect to any approach that nurtures striving towards personal gain without any regard to others.

Conversely, there are many people in this world who completely give of themselves and are always putting others' needs before their own. And then they wonder why they're not as happy or successful as they'd like to be!

There also seems to be an unhealthy balance of striving towards the achievement of material wealth or status, rather than being happy or being of service to others.

But your success is dependent upon others to some extent: whether they give you love, guidance or support, acceptance, provide services, help you, share resources, vote for you, or buy from you. Someone who is mindful of the needs and desires of others, and focuses on satisfying these, will enjoy more meaningful connections and benefit from their kindness in the long-term.

As well as being dependent upon others, do we not all also have a responsibility to fellow living creatures and the planet we're inhabiting?

To me, making a difference is about finding the right balance between doing what will make a difference to you and what makes a difference to others.

And if you ever doubt whether you as an individual have the ability to make a difference you'd love to make, consider the life of the young African village boy who became the incredible legacy of Nelson Mandela. Or those such as Adolf Hitler, who had such a horrific impact on so many people's lives. Everyone who has inspired you and been an influential change agent in the world (good or bad), started in the same way as you – an embryo in his or her mother's womb. And many of those who have had the greatest positive impact on the world grew up in environments that were not conducive to success. They will also have had lots of doubts and challenges along the way.

I love the quote by the Dalai Lama: 'If you think you're too small to make a difference, try going to bed with a mosquito.'[26]

A common 20th Century paradigm in Western workplaces was that the role of managers or leaders was to 'tell' those reporting to them what to do (based on the premise that staff were there to serve them). The concept of a leader's role including being of service to their people was a rarity. Many in senior positions enjoyed applying an authoritarian approach and feeding their egos so they could benefit personally from their team's efforts.

A concern frequently expressed by attendees of my leadership programmes is that they don't want to have to be someone they are not – someone who doesn't appear to care about others, or who displays behaviours that conflict with their values. Consistently they are so relieved to hear that being authentic and seeking to be of service to their teams is not only an acceptable approach to leading people, but is one that can yield better results.

In his book *Give And Take*, Professor Adam Grant shares fascinating findings from his research across different industries – that 'givers' are the best performers, averaging fifty percent more annual revenue than takers, who fall in the middle of the performance range. However *'givers dominate the bottom and top of the success ladder'[27]* so there are other aspects at play, too.

There can also be surprising by-products that come from 'giving' to others. Research shows that as well as adding meaning to your life, volunteering can help combat depression, make you happier, boost your confidence and self-worth, build a greater circle of friends and contacts, develop new skills, and advance your career. [28]

Personally, my whole life has transformed beyond recognition since I started being involved with Create Global Healing (the organisation I go to Rwanda with). I've found greater peace in myself because I now feel I have something of value to offer others, and the experiences I'm having can help put life's challenges into perspective. And my business has benefited in so many ways, too. Not only in terms of the focus and scope of my work, but

26 http://www.goodreads.com/quotes/7777-if-you-think-you-are-too-small-to-make-a

27 Give and Take, Adam Grant, Weidenfeld & Nicolson, 2013, p8

28 http://www.helpguide.org/life/volunteer_opportunities_benefits_volunteering.htm

also in the way my business continues to grow as a direct consequence of the humanitarian work and fundraising I do. And I now love teaching business owners how to grow their business by supporting a charity, too. So the ripple effect is happening.

So this principle is about making a difference, being of service, or doing what will help – in a way that your needs and those of others are met. It could be in terms of the 'big picture' – aligning your day-to-day activities with your life purpose or the legacy you want to leave in the world. Or making small changes that will make a difference to you or others.

The Giving Spectrum

Another way of thinking about 'making a difference' is in the context of giving, and what I call the 'giving spectrum':

• Imagine at one end of a spectrum there is **'unsustainable giving'** – this occurs when you love and respect others more than yourself; when you're kind to others but not to yourself; when you let others take advantage of you; or don't think that what you think or want is important (and so hold back on sharing this). The outcome of adopting this approach is that you may not be getting all your needs met; you may have unfulfilled dreams and aspirations; people may not treat you well; or you may be unhappy, knackered, stressed, or regularly ill because of all you're doing for others without looking after yourself. Others may perceive you as a kind soul or as a doormat.

• At the other end of the spectrum you have **'self-centred giving'** – this refers to people who adopt an approach where it's all about me, me, me! You'll know the kind – those who believe their needs, rights, and goals are far more important than those of others. And who demonstrate through their actions that caring about others is secondary to them or not important at all. Survival of the fittest is their motto, as they do what's important to them with little regard for others. This type of person is often perceived as unkind, arrogant, and selfish – with little apparent awareness of this.

• And in the middle is what I call **'strategic giving'** – this is one where naturally kind-hearted souls have learned how to adopt a healthy balance of loving and respecting themselves as well as others. When operating from here, you're connected to your heart and put yourself in the best place to succeed; you are making the difference you want to make in the world; you frequently enjoy success and good relationships; most of the time happiness, love, and gratitude ooze from your heart. You may be perceived as kind, happy, and successful.

And so applying this principle is about considering how you could make a difference to yourself as well as others, in a way that you have a healthy balance of:

- giving to yourself as well as others.

- making sure your own needs and desires are met in a way that is mindful of others.

- feeling good when you are both giving and receiving.

- being unconditional of your giving in the moment, whilst at the same time being assertive if your rights are violated.

- listening to your head AND your heart, and acting in alignment with this.

- setting positive intentions while being unattached to outcomes (see Chapter 17).

- applying all the heart values (love, kindness, compassion, integrity, respect, peace, and gratitude) that I discussed in previous chapters.

Knowing Your 'Why' – the Big Picture

When you are connected to your life or soul purpose, you're likely to feel more motivated to do what it takes to achieve your goals. And if you share your 'why' with others, you are also more likely to connect with like-minded souls, be more memorable, and attract more success.

Like the heart values in principle one, the concept is to work on yourself first and then to consider how you could have a positive impact on the lives of others.

Success becomes so much easier when you focus on your strengths, passions, and what's important to you (as I cover more in the next Chapter); when you master skills and a mind-set for success; and when you have a purpose in life that's bigger than you. For many, this purpose is bringing up a happy, healthy family, which without doubt is one of the greatest gifts you can give. However, if you want to be happy and energised when doing this (and avoid regrets or discontent later), it's also important to remain connected to your true authentic self.

Small Changes Can Make a Huge Difference

If you're someone who is motivated to make a difference, you may find yourself setting huge goals, putting too much pressure on yourself, and feeling overwhelmed. Doubts may also creep in – where do you start? Can you really make a difference? Is it really worth the effort?

But here's the thing: applying small changes consistently is a great way to get results. Especially if you like routines and are motivated when you are making progress (as you move forward with each step).

There are a couple of ways to do this:

1. Define a compelling, huge goal you'd love to achieve – then break it down into a series of small steps or things you could do each day or week, to take you to your goal.

OR

2. Decide what you could do differently each day – then work out the positive impact of doing this repeatedly over the long term. For example:

Saving £3 a day (e.g. by taking tea/coffee to work in a thermos mug rather than going to Starbucks) would give an extra £15 a week, £60 a month, and £720 a year – just think, what could you do with that?

Replacing a lunchtime sandwich with a healthy salad could save you 1750 calories (0.5lb) a week and knock 26lbs (almost 2 stone or 12 kgs) off your weight over a year. Is that so hard to do?

Calling one of your friends once a week could mean that you better keep in touch with those you love. Could these conversations enhance your life in any way?

Freeing up one hour a day to sit down and chat with your children while having dinner could transform your relationship with them now and for the rest of your lives. What's more important than that?

Every little change you make really can make a huge difference!

Making a Difference to Yourself

Do you ever get caught up in life? Feeling pressurised to keep others happy? Little time for you?

I find it fascinating that when asked 'how are you?' so many people in the Western world habitually say 'I'm really busy' – as though 'busyness' is the most important thing to be. As though 'busyness' is the only measure of success or worthiness. But is being busy really a measure of how you are? If you had a friend who wasn't busy, would you think any less of them or that they were unworthy of your friendship? Or could being able to turn off any feelings of 'busyness' and putting yourself in an emotional state of love and peace (rather than feeling the stress we often do when we're busy) enable you to be more effective in doing what really does need to be done?

Taking the time to reflect and pay attention to what your body, soul, and intuition tell you it's in your best interests to do, is a great way of being kind and compassionate to yourself.

What would make the biggest difference to you in the long term?

What is your body or intuition telling you it would be good for you to do today?

In most chapters of this book I share tools and techniques which you can use to make a difference to yourself. What I encourage you to do is not just to read this book, but to actually make a commitment to yourself, and to choose one thing that you could do each day to make a difference to YOU.

How could you increase the likelihood of doing this?

Making a Difference to Others

'The value of a man resides in what he gives and not in what he is capable of receiving.'

Albert Einstein

The scope of making a difference refers to your family, friends, community, and others you'd like to help or serve.

At the heart of making a difference to others is being of service to them in a way that helps them to get their needs met – without the need or goal of getting your needs met, too. That said, there are times when it will be appropriate to voice your needs and personal boundaries (e.g. the way you want to be treated). Or you may want to carry out voluntary activities to help plug a gap in your life, help you heal from a traumatic event, or to give your life more meaning – and that's fine, too.

Whether or not it's in your interest to serve more people just now will be dependent upon how much you already do this – remember BALANCE is an important aspect of 'making a difference'! If you're already running around doing too much for others at a cost to yourself, then I suggest you first take action that will put you in a better place physically, emotionally or spiritually. This could include considering whether it would be in your best interests to stop doing certain things for others.

If it feels 'right' to be making more of a difference to others, you could start by deciding to make a difference to one person each day – perhaps to set that intention and think about it several times a day until the opportunity arises, e.g. giving a compliment (when you mean it), carrying bags, stopping to help someone, giving someone your full attention, or asking how you could help someone.

Or you could make voluntary work part of your life – getting involved in a charity or community project. Sharing your skills and knowledge with others helps you recognise the value of what you've got to offer, may stimulate ideas or opportunities for change in other areas of your life, and help to build your skills and social network. Unpaid volunteers make a huge contribution to many communities and are often what helps glue them together.

When I decided to explore doing voluntary work, I knew there were several gaps in my life that I wanted it to fill: I would have loved to have had my own children – but for whatever reason this hadn't happened – and so I knew I wanted to spend time with young people; I used to feel useless when I saw film footage of refugees or those impacted by natural disasters or war, because I didn't have the skills of those who would fly out to help. So I wanted to use my skills to help those in critical need in some way; and with my number one passion being travel, I chose to get involved with a charity that enabled me to do more of this.

In Summary

A heart-centered approach to success includes being mindful of, and acting upon, what is really going to make a difference – to you and others. Your happiness and success is dependent upon having a healthy balance between giving to yourself and giving to others – embracing what I call 'strategic' giving. Effectively when you align your actions to what's really important to you and the impact you'd love to have, and remember to be kind to yourself, too, you will feel good and enjoy more meaningful success rather than finding the success you were striving for doesn't bring you happiness.

Resourceful Questions

Sometimes just asking yourself a question in a slightly different way will trigger new ideas:

• What would you like to say about your life when you're 80?

• What one thing could you do to improve your life today?

• What gaps do you have in your life that you could fill through voluntary work?

• How could you spend more time with your friends or family?

• What type of work would be better aligned to your values?

Empowering Affirmations

• I love that my work is aligned to the difference I want to make in the world.

• I have a lot to offer others in the world.

• What I do makes a difference.

• I have a good balance between looking after myself and serving others.

Tapping 'Set Up' Statements

• Even though I don't know what my life or soul purpose is yet, I deeply and completely love and accept myself.

• Even though I tend to 'give' to others more than myself, I know I can create a better balance

• Even though I don't know which cause I'd like to support, I know I'm in the perfect place to explore this.

Recommended Resources

• *Give and Take* by Adam Grant

• CSV Make A Difference Charity - http://www.csv.org.uk

• #givingtuesday (global day of giving to and supporting charities) – www.givingtuesday.org.uk or http://www.givingtuesday.org

Your Invitation To Inspire Others

I'd love to hear your experiences of helping others through any voluntary work you do and of any inspiration you've taken from this book.

Check out www.alisoun.com/heartude to find out how you can connect and find other resources that may help you.

Chapter 13

Principle 3 – Be The Masterful Authentic Leader You Were Born To Be

Proactively enhance your self-awareness and personal development to enable you to achieve results aligned to who you truly are, to have the greatest positive impact, and to inspire others to do the same.

I remember a few years ago babysitting for one of my nephews, and being surprised by the wisdom of this cute two-year-old. We were sitting on the sofa cuddled into one another as I read one of the *Thomas The Tank Engine* stories to him. As is often the case when reading to young children, there was a lot more discussion about the pictures in the book than the written text itself. On one page, I pointed at a picture and asked: 'What's different about that engine?' His response was simply, 'He's not different, he's special.' I was taken aback by the wisdom of this young soul for a few minutes, until we got to the end of the book and I realised that celebrating your uniqueness was the theme of the book!

Many children's fairy tales have a central character on a journey of personal discovery, including The Ugly Duckling, The Wizard Of Oz and Harry Potter. Have you ever felt you've more to offer or aren't happy with the life *you're* living? Perhaps you've drifted away from the true essence of who you are, or don't know even who that is any more.

Whatever your situation today, you have a special range of knowledge, skills, qualities, and talents – your unique gifts – even if you're not sure what these are right now. In the busy lives we've created in modern society, many people spend their time running around doing what they think they 'should' be doing or what they feel 'needs' to be done to survive in the world they have created for themselves. Often they've lost sight of what they're naturally good at, don't know what makes them unique, what they love, what excites them or makes them tick.

Their focus has become earning enough money to pay for clothes, childcare, the mortgage, holidays, and perceived necessities, often at the expense of their happiness and health. However, doing so much, spending too much time in stressful jobs (especially those you don't like), or compromising your values, is not sustainable.

'Success comes from knowing that you did your best to become the best that you are capable of becoming.'

John Wooden, Basketball Coach

I spent years striving for success in an industry that was killing my soul, and wondered why it felt like I was dragging my feet through wet concrete in an alien world. Why did I talk down my job when people asked me what I did? Why did I have this inner conflict of wanting to do well at my work while at the same time cringe at the thought of becoming the director of an investment company? It's only now, over a decade later, that I realise it was always going to be that way as long as I worked in that industry – because I couldn't get excited about making rich people richer when so many people in the world are suffering. Yes, I met lots of wonderful people in that world (many of whom I'm so grateful to still have as friends), but serving others with love, kindness, and compassion in that arena didn't appear to be as important as rewarding financial performance.

I was so relieved to wake up and realise in my mid-thirties that there was still plenty time to change the direction of my career. I still had more of my adult working life ahead of me than I'd lived, and therefore there was hope I could succeed and be happy by being and doing something else.

In order to enjoy authentic heart-centered success, there are a few foundations to put in place:

• **Knowing who you are** – otherwise how can you be authentic to this?

• **Knowing what you want** – so you can focus your attention on manifesting this.

• **Having a purpose, vision, and goals** – so you can add meaning and momentum to what you do.

Some people discover their purpose very early on in life, but for many they only explore this once they've become dissatisfied in some way with their life.

This chapter will give you ideas to help you recognise what makes you unique and to clarify your purpose. Then you can create the mind-set, emotional capacity, and action plan to support this.

There are two stages to becoming the best authentic leader you were born to be: *Self-awareness* – being clear on where you are now: your wants, needs and desires; which of your skills, talents and attributes you want to use; weaknesses; values and motivations, etc. *Personal Mastery* – come up with a compelling vision, goals, and plan to keep you on track for creating a happy and successful life that's aligned to your authentic best version of yourself. I've created a simple 7-step process for you to follow whenever you want to do this:

1. Identify what makes you unique in that situation.
2. Get clear on your purpose.
3. Create a compelling vision.
4. Define an exciting goal aligned to this.
5. Plan to make it happen.
6. Overcome any beliefs or feelings limiting your success.
7. Take inspired action!

Let's look at each of these in turn:

1. Identify What Makes You Unique

A great way to start exploring this is to ask yourself a whole range of resourceful questions:

Who am I?

Often people start answering this question by recounting the roles they have in life – as a parent, child, sibling, spouse, partner, friend, your job title, or what you do. And while these may be important relationships, you are far more than any one of these. How else would you define yourself?

- What skills and talents do you have?
- What do you love doing?
- What are you passionate about?

- How do you connect with others?

- What positive personal qualities and traits do you have?

- What is important to you (your values)?

- What motivates you?

- What do others compliment you on or say about you (your personal brand)?

- What makes you stand out?

- What do you stand for?

We are all multi-dimensional beings – you are your body, your mind, your soul, and your unique personal energy.

Being a collection of thoughts and feelings, how you define your identity influences what you do and what you'll manifest. Who you are today has been shaped by what you've thought until now. But both your mind and body have the power to re-create themselves, and that means you can create a whole different future for yourself, if you want to and decide to.

What am I good at?

It's easier to succeed and enjoy a happier, more rewarding life when you focus on what you love to do and what you naturally do well. While in most jobs we may need to compromise on this to some extent, any time you spend trying to overcome weaknesses or working to turn them into strengths can cause unnecessary stress. And it is a waste of your own unique gifts and energy. Instead, where possible, focus on your talents and strengths that capture your heart. Others who are great at your weaknesses can support you in these areas.

To identify your **strengths & passions:**

- Consider all the roles you play in life and list all the skills, strengths, and personal qualities you display in each of these. Remember the skills and talents you enjoyed as a child. Think about some of the most memorable things you've achieved in your life or you love doing.

- Ask others for feedback – often our friends, family, and colleagues see good qualities in us that we don't recognise.

- Be open to the possibility that you will have lots of talents you've just not discovered yet! Mind map or list all the things you'd love to try and then give them a shot.

One of my friends, Julie, is a wonderful example of someone who has benefited greatly from doing this. After a successful corporate career, Julie decided to change direction so she could manage her working hours around bringing up her young family. She decided to attend workshops on topics she was curious about. It was during one of these (a Theta Healing course) that two people completely independently of one another asked whether she'd ever considered making silver jewellery. This hadn't ever been something Julie had done, but trusting her instincts she signed up to a silver jewellery-making class. And within a few weeks she had set up a new business selling her work. Now, a couple of years later, she has a thriving business she loves and which means she has plenty of time for her family, too – all based on developing new creative skills she didn't know she had.

Here are my top three resources to help you identify your strengths:

· *Gallup Strength Finder 2.0* by Tom Rath – this is a great little book which gives you access to an on-line assessment and downloadable report that gives you feedback on your natural strengths and how to apply these.

· *Wealth Dynamics Report* – an excellent personalised report you can get on-line that gives insights into your natural path to success and financial abundance.

· *DISC Reports* – these reports, which you can again do on-line, give incredibly accurate insights into your natural and adapted behavioural styles.

What do I need?

It is natural to have needs and wants. Becoming a masterful authentic leader, however, involves being savvy in determining which of your needs to meet, desires to fulfil, and taking action to make this happen.

It's easier to manifest your desires and achieve your goals when your personal needs are being met. These could relate to survival (food, water, sleep, and a roof over your head); safety; health; social acceptance; to be loved and to love; social interaction; opportunities to learn; financial needs; or a sense of connection. Ask yourself:

• What do I <u>need</u> to survive?

• What do I need to grow and flourish?

• What do I need to let go of?

What do I want?

Once you've worked out a way to have your needs met, open up your creative mind to the abundance flow of possibilities and what you want:

- What dreams or desires do you have?
- What would you like to be part of?
- How would you like to feel?
- What brings you joy?
- What does your heart yearn for?
- What would make a difference to you?
- What makes you feel good?
- What do you feel you are missing in your life?

What motivates me (to take action)?

Consider your motivations then align the strategies for achieving your goal to these, to increase the likelihood that you'll start and remain focused on working towards it:

- What's important to you (your values)?
- What inspires you?
- What helps you succeed?
- What makes you feel good?

2. Get Clear on Your Purpose

Your purpose is the big picture that gives your life meaning, e.g. your family, what's important to you, or a cause close to your heart. It's what drives you and compels you to move forward towards your beacon in the darkness or divine light.

> 'Having a sense of purpose, having that sense of clarity, is I think what brings out the best in you and enables you to do the things you really want to do. And I think finding your place in society, finding your place in the world is absolutely key to this.'[29]

James Caan, Entrepreneur

Some people interpret this as 'life' purpose – what they are here to do in their lifetime; the legacy they'd like to leave in the world, which is often shaped by life experiences.

29 *Choice Point, Align Your Purpose, Harry Massey & Dr David Hamilton Phd, Hay House, 2011, p78*

Others have more of a spiritual interpretation of purpose – that it's your life force that existed before you were born, and continues in spirit after you've left this physical world, the part of you that's always there, even when you are unsure of who you are and when you doubt yourself. You may call this your soul, pure unconditional love, or your infinite or higher self. It's your inner guide that knows what's right for you in life. And, if all is not right, it gives you feedback through your body in the form of intuition, negative feelings, and physical sensations.

A few people have great clarity about their purpose, but many people are unsure what this is, so here are some ideas on how you can identify your purpose:

- If you like to make a difference, take the time to read and consider what I suggest in the last chapter.

- Listen to guided visualisations – there are many brilliant visualisations you can do to stimulate heartfelt ideas around your life or soul purpose.

- Meditate – you could meditate on any questions I've shared in this or the last chapter, or setting the intention of gaining clarity about your purpose before meditating and noticing what comes up. By meditating regularly (and listening to messages you receive), you increase your awareness and intuition, and make wiser choices that are aligned to what's in your highest good.

If you're struggling to connect with your purpose, please be reassured that many people find this a challenge. This is often the case for those who've been caught up in the rat race of life and have been disconnected from the essence of who they are for some time. For many people, the clarity of purpose only comes when they decide to make a change in their life and embrace their journey of personal discovery, e.g. start taking action to change something about their life. You can do this today by committing to do whatever resonates with you the most in this book. Be patient and trust your purpose will become apparent at a time that's right for you. Enjoy the process and see what unfolds for you –there are plenty of people and resources who can help you work this out.

3. Create a Compelling Vision

Imagine your life three years from now...

- What will you be spending your time doing?

- Who will you be spending your time with?
- What work will you be doing?
- How do you spend your free time?
- How are you serving others?
- What will you have achieved?
- Who will you have helped?

To get ideas:

- Consider who/what inspires you, and why? e.g. people, stories/pictures in magazines, books, films, TV programmes, etc.
- Create a vision board/scrap book/collage – this is a fabulous way to come up with ideas for creating a compelling vision and visual image of your ideal life – using pictures from your favourite magazines, travel brochures, leaflets, posters and photos, etc.
- To do this, set aside a couple of hours in a special place, and cut out all the pictures and phrases that appeal to you. Then collate these into a collage of your ideal life – who you'd like to be, where you'd like to go, what hobbies you'd have, relationships and family you'd have, the fun times, how you'd like to feel, and inspirational quotes.
- And, of course, once you've made this, put it somewhere you can see it every day to keep all your ideas alive and to help motivate you.

4. Define an Exciting Goal

Having a clear idea of what you want to achieve, keeping this at the fore-front of your mind and taking action aligned to this, is critical for success. Those who set themselves compelling goals connected to their vision are more likely to succeed – as long as their thoughts, feelings, and actions are aligned to these!

I'll be covering how to develop the mind-set and emotional capacity for success later, so let's just look at the principle of goal setting here.

Goal setting involves breaking your vision down into smaller bite-size goals, e.g. if your vision is to be in business for yourself, to enjoy a particular career, or complete a particular challenge, you're more likely to achieve this if you break this down into smaller goals for the next week, month, six months, or year.

I like to enjoy life and encourage others to do the same. So when considering your goals, choose ones that are going to make you feel good when you achieve them. And make them so compelling that you will do whatever it takes to succeed, no matter what.

Coming up with a compelling goal links in to what motivates you. One way to look at this is to consider whether you are an 'away from' or 'towards' person. I know I'm most likely to remain focused and take aligned action if I make the goal so big that it's exciting, or if I want to avoid a negative outcome.

I remember a few years ago a friend and I decided that we wanted to lose weight. We both knew we were more likely to achieve our goal if we put in place something to motivate us. Both being people who are 'away from' motivated people, we decided to come up with forfeits that would apply if we didn't achieve our goals. As a vegan and Chief Executive of an animal rights charity, it was easy for my friend. She gave me a cheque for £50 that I was to send to an organisation which carried out experiments on animals – something that clashed so much with what she was about at a core level; so a really strong motivator. For me, it wasn't so easy. After a couple of hours, she suggested that if I didn't meet my goal, she would post a photo of me naked on the Internet. I can still feel the knot in my stomach as I think about this – it wouldn't be good for anyone! And, boy, did I make sure I achieved my goal, with far more focus and ease than when I've not aligned my goals to strong personal motivations.

When setting your goals, I suggest you define these using the following 'SMARTA' format:

- **Specific** – your goal is detailed enough to know what you're working towards, e.g. 'to have published and sold 100 copies of my first Kindle book' is more specific than 'to have published my first book'.

- **Measureable** – there is a clear way you can measure your progress/ results.

- **Achievable** – you have the resources to make this happen (time, money, and whatever else you need).

- **Relevant** – aligned to your vision and what's important to you.

- **Time bound** – remember to have short-term goals that feed into your big goal (e.g. goals on the same topic for one month, six months, and one year). And goals with specific deadlines (e.g. 31/12/14) rather than the vagueness of 'this year'.

- **Action** – consider how you could make your goal more compelling or exciting, so you're motivated to only take action that will help you achieve it.

5. Plan to Make it Happen

Create an action plan to keep you focused – putting in place what you need to achieve your goal, including scheduling tasks or activities into your diary, and gathering all the resources you need. You may find this more compelling if you do this kind of planning somewhere that will inspire you – either in a room in your home that you've 'furnished' to nurture your creativity, or somewhere else. There's a hotel near me on the beach that I love to go and work from. Depending on your goal, there are lots of mobile apps available to help you keep focussed, motivated, and to monitor your progress.

6. Overcome any Beliefs or Feelings Limiting Your Success

Identify any doubts, fears, or negative feelings in relation to your goal, and take action to overcome these. This is a critical step that most people miss – you can find out more about how to do this in Chapters 15 and 16.

7. Take Inspired Action

Follow your plan! And remember to do what it takes to remain motivated to do this including sharing your progress with others if this keeps you engaged.

In Summary

You are more likely to live the life you'd love to live or to enjoy success when you are proactive in taking action to discover your life purpose and revolve your life around this. Those who achieve their dreams are masters at applying a process similar to the one I've shared in this chapter.

I regularly take time out to consider what goals I want to achieve in the next six months or year, and take myself through the process I've shared above. Sometimes I achieve them, and sometimes I don't. I'm motivated by setting myself huge goals, and so even if I don't achieve them I know I've got nearer my dreams than if I had not set the goal or if I'd set small goals which wouldn't have been exciting enough.

Writing this book has been a goal of mine for the last couple of years, and the fact that you're reading it means that I've achieved my goal. It may have taken longer than I'd anticipated at the start but I know the content is so much better because of what I've experienced until now.

Resourceful Questions

• How could you be the best person you were born to be?

• What one thing would you love to achieve this year?

• What would you like others to say about your life when you're 80?

Affirmations

• It's great to be successful just being me!

• I'm so grateful for the life I've created for myself.

• I love what I do every day.

• I love living the life I was born to have.

Tapping 'Set Up' Statements

• Even though I've no idea who I am, I deeply and completely love myself, forgive myself, and accept myself.

• Even though I don't feel I have anything to offer, I deeply and completely love myself, forgive myself, and accept myself.

• Even though I don't know what the future holds, I know I'll be OK.

• Even though I find making changes scary, I know I'll be fine.

Recommended Resources

• Gallup Strength Finder 2.0 by Tom Rath

• Wealth Dynamics Report - http://wdprofiletest.com/

• Enneagram Personality Reports - http://www.enneagraminstitute.com/

• Various reports profiling reports about happiness and your values – www.authentichappiness.com

• DISC Behavioural Profiles

• *Discover What You're Here To Do* by Nicola Grace

- *Screw Work Let's Play* by John Williams
- *The Path To Transformation* by Shakti Gawain

Chapter 14

Principle 4 – Embrace Personal Leadership & Responsibility

Proactively direct your life by taking responsibility for choosing thoughts, feelings and actions that will enable you to enjoy more meaningful success and inspire others to be the best they can be, too.

Has there ever been a time when you've felt stressed, worried or anxious about something that is out of your control, blamed others or situations for what's not going well for you, or felt that life isn't fair?

I've been delivering Personal Leadership & Responsibility workshops in workplaces for a few years now, and participants often say it's such a relief and so empowering to discover that they can choose how they respond to situations around them. They are delighted to learn that there is the potential for them to achieve their desired outcomes if they focus on consciously taking action aligned to these.

I often start these workshops by asking attendees to come up with the personal qualities they'd be looking for if they were responsible for selecting people to complete a specific task or activity, e.g. at home, at work, or in their communities.

Consistently, the type of people they say they like to employ, spend time with, or buy from, are those who are kind, friendly, generous, trustworthy, hardworking, fun, positive, considerate, skilled, solution-focussed or proactive. I've never had any group say they'd take on negative, moaning, unskilled, problem-focussed, self-centred, lazy or unreliable people. And yet, I'm sure you'll know plenty of people who are this way, who constantly blame everything else and everybody else for what's not going well in their lives, not realising they are making things harder for themselves than need be and are hindering their own success.

Now don't get me wrong. Life throws some awful curve balls at us every so often, and it's healthy to experience a full spectrum of emotions – both positive and negative – in response to life's events, particularly when you're in the early stages of coping with a situation that triggers intense feelings of shock, grief, trauma or loss. The application of this principle relates to how you take responsibility for responding to less acute situations (or once an appropriate period of time has lapsed since a traumatic event). Or the approach you take to be successful.

I can't think of anything worse than losing loved ones, being seriously ill, abused, injured, raped, homeless, penniless, or witnessing the atrocities of war. One of these experiences would be bad enough, but sadly these are typical experiences of those we support in Rwanda. And yet, like many others who have endured horrors most of us would not want to even imagine, the young people we've been working with have taught me the human body's capacity to heal. They've shown me that when you have nothing, you either step into a sense of responsibility for doing what you can to survive – or you die.

Tragically, it is that critical for many people in this world, and so many do die because the resources they need are not available, through no fault of their own. But what inspires me are all those who, despite going through some of the worst situations we could ever face as human beings, are able to call on their inner strength, to be happy again, and to create a better future for themselves than they would if they chose to play the victim.

It's Your Choice

You see, it's not what happens to you that determines how you feel, but how you choose to act in situations, based on the skills and resources available to you at any given time.

In most situations, you do have a choice – to take responsibility for the part you play in reaction to events around you – the way you create opportunities for yourself, or blame others and events for how you're feeling and what's happening 'to' you. In other words, you can choose to focus on either the positive or negative aspects of a situation – each moment is a choice point:

• to think solely of yourself, or to consider others

• to act, or to do nothing

• to embrace life with all its ups and downs, or to play the victim

• to create new possibilities, or to stay in your comfort zone.

The way you choose to respond to events (albeit often at an unconscious level) will determine both how you feel on a day-to-day basis and the results you get.

'There are three constants in life… change, choice and principles.'

Stephen Covey

Take Responsibility	Avoid Responsibility (blame)
– Usually express positive thoughts, emotions and/or behaviours	– Often express negative thoughts, emotions and/or behaviours – moaning & complaining
– Often take healthy and appropriate steps to best cope with life's challenges	– Have a negative approach – blaming others or events for not getting desired results
– Have a positive proactive 'I can do /I can learn' attitude	– Don't take action to help themselves – either doing nothing or adopting unhealthy habits
– Present reasons for things going well or not	– Present 'excuses' for when things don't go well
– Focus on solutions/what could work/planning	– Focus on problems/what's not working/the past
– Admit to and learn from successes/mistakes	– Don't accept responsibility for, nor learn from mistakes
– Create and embrace opportunities	– Like to stay within their comfort zone
– Work hard & are reliable	– Do the minimum & are unreliable
More likely to succeed (if also technically competent)	**Less likely to succeed (even if technically competent)**

When we act responsibly, we feel we have a choice and are more likely to demonstrate positive, proactive and solution-focused behaviours, e.g. acting with love, peace, and compassion in our hearts, managing our emotions effectively, and embracing an abundance-based mentality. Those who consistently adopt this approach are often more likely to be happier, healthier, enjoy loving relationships, and to succeed in life. They will naturally attract others like them, they may be popular and push themselves outside their comfort zone in a quest to make the most of life. When things go wrong, they find healthy ways to cope and become more resilient.

The alternative approach is to focus on what's wrong or not working, who or what is to blame for a situation you find yourself in, or to focus on what you perceive as problems and do nothing about resolving the situation. Have you ever noticed that some people have an endless supply of excuses as to why they 'can't' do something? Or you maybe know people who usually come across as angry, negative, or defensive? Sadly, yet not unsurprisingly, people who adopt this kind of approach are more likely to spend a lot of their time unhappy and unhealthy. When in this emotional place, we feel we have no choice but to tolerate what's happening. This isn't a pleasant place to be. If you ever feel this way, please be assured that there is usually something you can do to improve your situation, including seeking the help or support of someone who could help you. While I'm a great proponent of natural remedies, there are times when taking prescribed drugs may be the best solution in the short-term, until you work out whether something else could work better for you.

Language such as 'it's not my fault' or 'I'm like this because of my mum/dad' are obvious giveaways of someone who is not taking responsibility for what's going on in their life. They may present these responses as reasons for a particular outcome, but they really are excuses, as they infer blame rather than any sense of ownership.

Sometimes people find it difficult to take on the suggestion that you can choose how to respond to events, particularly when someone has done something cruel or unpleasant to them, or it is easier to blame circumstances. So let's be clear, this isn't about taking responsibility for something others do to you, nor pretending that all is well or 'fair' in the world. It's about choosing how you respond to all situations, good or bad. When things don't go as you'd like, you can either wallow in self-pity, complain or moan but take no positive action. Or you can acknowledge how you feel and then take conscious positive action to put yourself in a better position.

Taking responsibility is not about blaming yourself, either. When we apportion blame, we are being critical rather than loving. It's far healthier to recognise and accept the part you've played in creating whatever you're experiencing, from a place of self-love and acceptance that you always do the best you can in any moment. Yes, with hindsight or more life experience, you might now choose to act differently, but you always do the best you can with the resources available to you.

Nor is taking responsibility about blaming others – in the same way, you can only do the best you can with what you know and the resources you have available in any moment. That is the same for others, too. Everyone works with their own awareness at any given time.

Your Genes Don't Always Control Your Health

Our health is one area of life where science is beginning to prove we have more influence than we used to think. Many of us have been programmed with the belief that genes control our health and that we are victims of the biology we've inherited from our parents. However, the science of epigenetics undermines this theory, as it proves that the environments we expose our bodies to also influence our health. In other words, we no longer need to be the victim of our genes – we may inherit genetic blueprints that influence our traits, personality, and health, but we can also influence our reality by changing the environments we put our bodies into, e.g. what we eat, what we feel, the toxins we expose ourselves to, and how we choose to help ourselves recover when we get ill (either physically, emotionally or mentally).

'The science of epigenetics, which literally means "control above genes" profoundly changes our understanding of how life is controlled.'[30]

Dr Bruce Lipton, Renowned Cell Biologist

We may have learned unhealthy habits or coping strategies when we were young, which we can change if we choose to. In the same way, we can change beliefs and behaviours that no longer serve us, if we choose to.

I've often believed that I'm not built to run marathons, but the English long distance runner Steve Way has inspired me to consider this may not be the case. A former 16½-stone (105kg) couch potato who drank and smoked heavily, Steve decided to turn his life around in 2007 and has since achieved the amazing feat of breaking a UK record and coming tenth in the 2014 Commonwealth Games Marathon. We all have that capacity for creating a

---

30 Bruce H. Lipton, PHD, The Biology Of Belief, 2008, Hay House, p37

better future for ourselves, and for others.

Of course it's human for even the most positive of people to feel low or challenged. And there may be situations where you find it easy to take responsibility, but others where you revert into more 'childlike' behaviours and tendencies.

What I suggest (and discuss further in the next chapter) is to pay attention to what you feel and to use your body as a feedback mechanism on whether or not it would be beneficial for you to think, feel, and act differently.

I know I've been very fortunate in the way that most of my life experiences have led me to be very positive, optimistic, and proactive. However, there are times where I can find myself feeling more challenged in being able to maintain a positive, 'responsible' approach. But I know that's OK, because I know I'm human and I've learned tools and techniques to help me pick myself up, feel calm, or positive again more quickly.

Most positive people prefer to spend time with, to work with, and to buy from someone who is kind, generous, positive, proactive, enthusiastic, and solution-focused. People often feel drained by those who are negative, needy, or bitchy most of the time.

Likewise, negative people who complain, find fault, are critical, or gossip, attract like-minded friends and experiences, because they can relate better to each other and keep each others' woes alive.

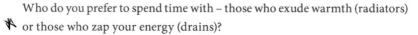

Who do you prefer to spend time with – those who exude warmth (radiators) or those who zap your energy (drains)?

You are Shaping Your Reality

Remember that who you attract is a reflection of the way you are being. And that's great if those around you are those you want to have in your life. However, if you're attracting lots of negative, angry, fearful or miserable people in your life, consider how you are being that way, too. Remember, of course, to recognise that we all have ups and downs – so it's not a case of eliminating all negative people from your life but to be conscious of who you are allowing in and to support those you want in your life when they need it.

There is no right or wrong; it's a choice. But if you want to be happy, healthy, and successful, you will make this easier on yourself in the long-run if you begin taking responsibility for thinking, feeling, and acting in a way that's aligned to heart-centered success. That's because what you think has an impact on what you feel. What you feel has an impact on what you do. And what you do has an impact on the results that you get. This includes who you choose to spend time with, what skills you decide to learn, and how you choose to cope with challenges you face.

Personal responsibility also extends into taking responsibility for the part you play in creating the outcomes or changes you want to see in your life and the world. Have you ever heard people advocating peace in the world who are not particularly peaceful or loving towards those they live or work with? Often they are totally unaware they are the initiators of conflict in their lives, and don't realise that by simply changing their own approach, they could obtain completely different responses from those around them.

Which of the following approaches do you think would be most likely to elicit positive outcomes (feelings, results or responses)?

- Trying to get children to bed by screaming at them versus being loving towards them?

- Telling a partner how they annoy you versus what you love about them?

- Focussing on what you don't like versus what you do like?

- Spending hours talking about a problem versus finding a solution?

- Drinking or eating excessively to make yourself feel better versus participating in a healthier activity?

Often people are not aware of the incongruence between their desired outcomes or impact and others' perceptions of their actions.

I remember meeting someone who trained business owners on how not to be a pushy salesperson, and yet her daily bombardment of promotional emails about this led me to form the opinion that she was both pushy and not someone I'd do business with. I'm sure she was doing the best she could, but I'm not sure she got many takers on her courses!

Take a moment just now to consider:

- What approach you take – do you usually take responsibility, or avoid it?

- Are you happy with the results you are getting in life?

- Is there scope for you to take more responsibility in any area of life?

Please congratulate yourself on all the good that you are manifesting for you and for those around you!

And for anything that's not going the way you'd like, contemplate how you could turn the situation around.

Another factor that will help is to have an awareness of whether you are focussing on what you can or cannot control. Often when we feel stressed, anxious or worried, we are placing our attention on what we can't control about a situation and so it's no wonder we don't feel good or are disappointed with the results we get. However, you will feel better and get improved results by shifting your focus to what you can control in the situation (e.g. what you think, feel, and do) and then taking action aligned to this.

Playing the Lead Role in Your Life

Whenever you feel challenged, don't like what you're experiencing, or want to make a change in your life, there's a very simple series of questions that you can ask yourself to help you decide what to focus on. These have helped me work out the best way forward on many occasions, and I know they have really helped many of my clients, too. All you do is ask yourself each of these questions, in this order:

1. What part have I played in creating this situation? What part could I play in getting the result I'd like?

There will be a part you play in most situations – what you think, feel, do, and how you act.

2. In this situation what CAN you control or influence?

In any situation, all you can control (or learn to control) is what you think, feel, do, and how you do it.

3. In this situation, what can you NOT control or influence?

You obviously can't control how others think, feel, and the action they take, but you can often influence them.

4. How could you best respond to this situation?

In a way that meets your values and puts you in the best place to succeed.

In Summary

Personal leadership and responsibility is about recognising the part you play in how you feel and the results you get; consciously choosing to interact positively with events/people around you; and taking action aligned to this. For example:

- treating others with love, kindness and compassion

- proactively managing your emotions effectively

- doing what you can to make a difference

- stepping into being the best that you can be

- committing to learning what will help you be happy and successful

- making the most of opportunities that present themselves

As with many of the principles I'm sharing with you in this book, the first stage is to turn off the autopilot and be more consciously aware of your feelings so that you can use these as a barometer for whether or not you need to take any remedial action. I cover this more in Chapters 15 & 17.

Resourceful Questions

Be really honest and ask yourself the following questions about how you could take more responsibility:

- What part have I played in creating this situation (that I don't like)?

- In this situation, what CAN I control?

- In this situation, what CAN'T I control?

- What would be the best way to respond to this?

- How could I take more responsibility for XXX (e.g. my happiness or success)?

Empowering Affirmations

- I feel better when I focus on what I can control, and let go of what I can't.

- I know I can create an abundance of success.

- It's great to feel more in control again.

- I love making things happen.

- When 'bad' things happen, I do my best to cope.

Tapping 'Set Up' Statements

- Even though I don't like XXX, I accept I had a part to play in creating this outcome.

- Even though I'm not sure how I can feel better/get better results, I deeply and completely accept myself.

- Even though I don't think it was my fault, I am open to exploring what part I played in this.

Recommended Resources

- *The Soul Of Leadership* by Deepak Chopra

- *The Seven Habits Of Highly Effective People* by Stephen Covey

- *The Biology Of Belief* By Bruce Lipton

- *Managing Brand You* by Jerry S. Wilson & Ira Blumenthal

Chapter 15

Principle 5 – Manage Your Emotions

Manage your emotions effectively so you can choose to respond calmly to challenges; channel your energy towards the things you can control, so you can create the best potential outcomes for you and those around you.

One of the most remarkable women I know is the author Kim Macleod, who wrote an incredibly moving and inspiring book, *From Heartbreak To Happiness*. With admirable bravery and honesty, Kim shares her journey of not only learning to cope with the tragic sudden death of her 12-year-old son Calum from meningitis, but also how she went on to teach others how to have more happiness in their lives through her Happiness Clubs.

In her book, she says, 'Making the choice to be happy, taking small steps, being patient and kind to myself, asking for help, letting go of emotion, finding my passion and deciding to follow it, are the strands that have knitted it together.'[31]

Knowing Kim, it's her positivity, warmth, and energy that stand out and transcend any doubts about whether we can heal emotional wounds and create a happy rewarding life for ourselves – if we choose to do so.

One of the reasons many of the young people we work with in Rwanda are now enjoying happy lives again is that, like Kim, instead of giving up or adopting a victim mentality, they also chose – after an appropriate amount of time – to let go of their trauma and stress, using healthy coping strategies. Most can still remember the events that they experienced during the genocide, but these memories no longer have the strong negative emotional charge once associated with them.

31 Kim Macleod, From Heartbreak To Happiness, Marplesi, 2013, p109.

In the same way that your brain and 'mindbody' can instantly create a reliable undesirable response to a situation (e.g. as happens to create phobias), it's also possible to quickly create lasting change, to neutralise negative emotions triggered by traumatic events.

What You Feel Matters When it Comes to Success

• Remember, it's your emotions that drive your actions and the results you get. So when you consciously set yourself a goal (e.g. relating to weight loss, money, health, your job, a business or sporting accomplishment), holding onto negative feelings such as stress, upset, depression, anxiety, nerves or unworthiness, will limit your success.

• And, as I explained in Chapter 3, positive and negative emotions trigger different chemical and biological reactions in your body. Your body has not yet evolved to be able to cope with long-term stress in an efficient or sustainable manner, so doing what you can to maintain a positive emotional state as much of the time as possible will improve your health and resilience to life events. You are also likely to be able to make better decisions.

• Whether or not you consciously choose to manage it, the way you feel is infectious and will be having an impact on how others around you feel. This, in turn, influences how they respond to you.

As Dr David Hamilton highlights in his book, *The Contagious Power of Thinking*, emotions spread just like physical viruses do – happiness is contagious, but so is depression. 'If a friend of yours has become depressed for any reason, it increases the likelihood that you will also become depressed by 93%.'[32] So wouldn't it be good if you could help them feel better by putting yourself in a good emotional state, as well as offering them support?

• Have you ever felt uplifted by being around others who are positive, enthusiastic or energised? Calm around calm people? Or felt your energy drain away when you're in the company of people who moan or complain all the time? Sustainable success depends on you enjoying good health and relationships, both of which are greatly influenced by your emotional state and ability to cope with life's challenges.

• How you feel around a pregnant woman even affects the emotional and

---

32 *The Contagious Power Of Thinking, Dr David R Hamilton PHD, Hay House, 2011, pX*

physical health of her unborn child. The science of epigenetics shows that the environment the foetus is in (influenced by how the mother feels and the resulting hormones pumping through her body), also affects how it will grow and be once born.

- Studies also show that the way leaders manage their emotions has an impact on the profitability of a business.

In this chapter, I'm going to share ways to change how you feel naturally – both in the moment, as well as hard-wiring your brain and mind for future resilience and success. Like many of the techniques I've already shared, typically these involve either deliberately putting yourself in a positive emotional state so you feel good, or taking action to overcome negative emotions when it is appropriate to do so.

Sometimes, when I suggest to attendees at my events that they can change how they feel, I am very quickly met with scepticism. And, to be perfectly honest, I felt that way, too, when first presented with this. Until then, I didn't know you could do this, nor did I understand the difference it could really make. I knew my life wasn't how I wanted it to be; there was something missing. I could feel a spark and glimmer of hope in my heart that I could create a happier and more satisfying life, but I didn't know how. And so I decided to give this a shot. Without doubt, that has been one of the best decisions I've ever made. And what I've since discovered, through my own personal experience and working with hundreds of clients over the years, is that – yes, in most day-to-day situations, it is possible to change what you think and feel.

I wonder if you've ever used any of the following coping strategies to change how you feel:

- having a glass of wine or beer?

- eating chocolate, sweets or cakes?

- having a cigarette?

- taking prescription or over-the-counter drugs?

- taking recreational drugs?

- going shopping?

If you have done any of these activities, you've already been managing your emotions, but while these can make you feel better in the short-term (and

I am partial to the odd glass of wine myself), they are often not sustainable – especially if you keep going back for more each time you need a lift. Long-term, these will cause you more harm than good.

Instead, what I'm sharing in this chapter are ways you can feel good which are healthy, natural, and sustainable – they can have a positive long-term impact on your health and how long you'll live. And they often don't cost you a penny, either!

I'm not saying that conventional pharmaceutical drugs don't work – often they do. And in some circumstances, they are the best solution. However, it deeply saddens me that so many people are suffering because they don't have enough tools in their tool kit to make themselves feel good naturally or that would work well alongside other medication.

While most people in developed countries enjoy much higher living standards than of 100 years ago, too many people are not happy:

- Between 8% and 12% of the UK population experience depression in any year. [33]

- The World Health Organisation forecasts that by 2020 depression will be the second leading contributor to the global burden of disease.[34]

- 59% of British adults say their life is more stressful than it was five years ago.[35]

- Approximately 30% of all consultations with doctors are related to a mental health problem.[36]

As I've mentioned before, as a human being it's important to feel the full spectrum of emotions – all the positive ones and the negative feelings (such as grief, loss, shock, fear and sadness) that are appropriate responses to life events. However, being able to choose to feel positive emotions and to let go

---

33 Mental Health Foundation, *The Fundamental Facts The latest facts and figures on mental health, 2007 Edition (ref Singleton N, Lewis G. Better Or Worse: A Longitudinal Study Of The Mental Health Of Adults Living In Private Households In Great Britain London: The Stationery Office pxviii, (2003))*

34 Mental Health Foundation, *The Fundamental Facts The latest facts and figures on mental health, 2007 Edition (ref 14 - The World Health Report 2001*
Mental Health: New Understanding, New Hope Geneva: World Health Organisation, (2001))

35 Mental Health Foundation Article, *Nearly half of adults feel stressed every day or every few days, 8 January 2013, http://www.mentalhealth.org.uk/our-news/news-archive/2013-news-archive/130108-stress/*

36 Mental Health Foundation, *The Fundamental Facts The latest facts and figures on mental health, 2007 Edition (ref 178 - Norwich Union, Health Of The Nation Index, at www.healthofthenation.com, (2004))*

of negative feelings that are no longer serving you (when it's appropriate), is healthy and empowering.

Knowing how to do this enables you to move forward in a way that is in your highest interest, rather than blocking out or numbing the upset or stress. Mental illness is one of the biggest challenges we face in modern society, because most people are not educated on how their mind and body works; how they can help themselves recover; and sometimes because they don't receive the professional support they need – often because many medical professionals are not trained on this either, or don't know enough about alternative interventions or complementary medicines.

'Our feelings are a feedback mechanism to us about whether we're on track or not.'

Jack Canfield, Author

We all have a part to play in helping ourselves and others to lead happier healthier lives. By learning to manage your emotions you'll then be impacting how others around you feel, and be able to be of greater support to others when they are suffering.

Managing How You Feel in The Moment

This is a bit like taking a paracetamol or aspirin when you have a headache – you take action to change how you feel in the moment. However, there may well be a root cause which is also worth tackling, e.g. having eaten or drunk something that doesn't agree with you, not being hydrated enough, or putting yourself under too much stress.

In 2003 I developed a powerful model with a good friend, Fiona Ogg, that forms the foundation of our Pure Happiness Course[37]. Participants love it because it provides a simple framework for remembering what they can do to change how they feel. And if you practise this advice regularly, you will be able to change how you feel in the moment and experience many long-term effects, too.

While some of the activities may seem basic, they really can make a huge difference when you consciously choose to do them to change how you feel.

I remember speaking at a conference for Bipolar sufferers and, before I delivered my presentation, being unsure if what I was about to share (the

---

37 See www.purehappiness.co.uk *or contact me through* www.alisoun.com *to find out more.*

same as what you'll read shortly) would really make a difference to those in the audience. I was therefore surprised and overwhelmed by the number of people who spoke to me afterwards about how uplifted they had felt. And even more so when I received many emails in the subsequent days and weeks from people who were feeling so much better because they were practising what they'd learned.

The Holistic SMILE

I can guarantee you'll already be doing some of what I'm about to share with you, though you may not realise the benefits of doing them:

1. S = Smile

This is one of the quickest and simplest things you can do to change how you feel, because when you smile, you physically send a message to your brain that instructs the release of a unique blend of chemicals in your body which make you feel good.

It's a bit like having a whole series of taps in your brain controlling the release of the different chemicals throughout your body. In order for you to feel stress, anxiety or fear, the right taps have to be turned on to pump the chemicals (such as adrenaline, cortisol and norepinephrine) you need in your body to feel those feelings. By contrast, when you feel good, other taps in your brain are turned on to release hormones such as endorphins and oxytocin.

Every feeling has a unique blend of chemicals which your body releases to enable you to feel each emotion. So to change how you feel, you effectively turn off the taps for stress, fear and anxiety, and turn on the taps for peace, calm or confidence. When you have more feel-good hormones pumping through your body more of the time, you're going to feel better. It's that simple.

You don't even have to feel happy when you smile – the act of smiling will trigger the chemical reaction in your body that will help lift your mood.

Another good thing about smiling is that it's contagious. We have mirror neurons in our brain that reflect back body language which we see in others. So when somebody smiles at you, you are programmed to smile back and vice versa (unless there are personal reasons not to). If someone smiles back at you, they will be releasing feel good hormones in their body, so you are literally helping the world become a happier place.

Smiling is also often perceived as an indicator that a person is friendly, approachable, happy, and confident – all endearing qualities that can help build connections, harmonious relationships, and create opportunities for success.

How often do you smile? When could you smile more?

2. M = Move

There are many benefits for moving, though what I'm going to focus on here is how movement and exercise can change how you feel, how others perceive you, and, consequently, the results you get.

Every single emotion you feel has a different posture associated with it. In other words, the way you stand, sit or walk has an impact on the way you feel.

The act of moving has a similar effect on the 'taps in your brain' which I mentioned earlier. By simply changing your posture, you send signals to your brain about the blend of chemicals you want it to release in your body.

Changing how you stand, sit or walk is one of the quickest ways you can change how you feel. So whenever you feel an emotion you don't want to feel, remember to change your physical posture to one that corresponds with how you'd like to feel. Sometimes the easiest way to do this is to simply ask yourself – how would I stand, sit or walk, if I was feeling, e.g. happy? Then physically move your body in response to your question. Hold this new posture, and after a few moments, notice how you feel.

Research studies increasingly show that regular physical exercise is a good way to overcome depression. A recent Mental Health Foundation (UK) survey found that 'a greater proportion of people who had tried exercise as a treatment for depression, found it effective (81%) than found anti-depressants effective (70%)'.[38] And yet only 5% of doctors prescribe exercise as one of their top three treatments for mild or moderate depression.[39]

From a success perspective, it's also worth considering how your body language (including your facial expressions and how you're standing or sitting) influences how other people respond to you. Have you ever met

---

38 *Exercise and depression – online survey results, Mental Health Foundation, (2005)*

39 *Up and Running? Exercise Therapy And The Treatment Of Mild or Moderate Depression In Primary Care London: Mental Health Foundation p8, (2005)*

anyone who was saying all the right things but there was just something about them you didn't trust, you weren't sure about them, or you just didn't believe what they were saying?

That's because only 7% of the way you interpret what others 'say' comes from their actual words; 38% of the interpretation comes from how they say the words (their tonality); and 55% is based on your interpretation of their body language. And if their body language or tonality conflicts with the words they're saying, then you simply won't believe the words.

But here is the challenge – your feelings automatically influence your body language and tonality. This is obviously fine if you are feeling good, confident, or another resourceful positive emotion. But if you doubt yourself, feel nervous or are anxious, others pick up on this from what you say, your body language, and tonality. And as a consequence, you may not get the results you are looking for. Would you take the advice of someone who appears to doubt what they are saying? Or go to dinner with someone who didn't appear to like you?

So managing your emotions effectively is not only important for your health and wellbeing, it also has a direct impact on how others perceive you and the results you get. Take time to reflect on how you're standing or sitting in a moment of distress, then change it to the way you'd stand or sit if you were feeling the way you'd love to feel (e.g. calm, confident or assertive). This is a great way to help you change how you feel there and then.

By moving more each day, you'll also improve your physical health, emotional resilience, and life expectancy. If exercise isn't yet something you enjoy or participate in every day, I suggest you consider what type of activity you could enjoy, how much time you've got available, and the specific outcomes you're looking for. For example, Tai Chi or Qigong are great for relaxation and spiritual development; walking 10,000 steps a day is a great general target for low impact fitness and can be fitted in to most lifestyles; something like yoga, ballet or Pilates is great for toning or flexibility; and dancing, running, swimming, cycling, or one of the many aerobic classes, are all great for weight loss. And, of course, you can also do good for others by joining in one of the many charity challenges you can find out about on-line.

3. I = Imagination

Your imagination really is one of the most powerful tools at your disposal because, when it comes to using your imagination, the brain doesn't know the difference between what you actually do and what you imagine yourself doing. In both cases, there are physical changes to the structure of your brain and how you feel.

When you do or imagine doing something, you create what are called neuro-pathways in your brain. It's a bit like going for a walk across a field of crops or snow. When you first walk across that field, you have to push your way through the snow or crops to create a path. But if you were to walk back and forth along the same section, you'd physically erode a path in that field. Then the next time you enter the field, you'd most likely follow the path of least resistance – the one you've been down before. And that is what effectively goes on in your brain, both when you physically do something again and again and again; and when you imagine yourself doing something again and again and again.

This is why visualisation is hugely popular in many sports, particularly by competitors at the top of their game, e.g. in athletics, golf, skiing, riding, tennis, and swimming. Gymnasts imagine performing perfect routines in their head before physically getting onto their apparatus. Golfers visualise where the ball is going to go. Hurdlers imagine running each pace between each hurdle, clearing them, running across the line with elation, and standing on the podium listening to their national anthem.

From a success perspective, it's important to understand the power of visualisation so that you can take control of the images and movies you play in your mind (which are manifestations of your thoughts). These images in your mind influence the results you get, in the same way as your audio thoughts do – negative images and self-talk both trigger negative emotions and limit your success.

Do you ever lie in bed at night worrying about what's coming up the next day? Because if you do, and you're playing movies of what could go wrong, you are physically creating connections in your brain which will influence what you do the following day. Running these movies in your mind triggers the release of the chemicals in your body which make you feel stressed or anxious – both in anticipation and during the event.

It would be far more effective for you to erase any destructive movies and to replace these instead with images of what you would like to happen.

Depending on the trigger that created the negative movie, you may need the help and support of someone who can take you though this, e.g. using techniques such as NLP, tapping or hypnotherapy. But one simple exercise you could practise for yourself is simply to mentally imagine and rehearse what you'd like to happen – a technique more commonly known as visualisation.

- **Mental Rehearsal Visualisation**

Simply visualising your desired outcomes doesn't guarantee you'll achieve these, as there will be many factors at play. But mastering this as a skill, and running your preferred movie several times in your head, will mean you feel better when anticipating what's coming up (rather than feeling stressed) and you'll be far more likely to perform better when the time comes. To do this, run through the event that's coming up in your mind (imagining you can see what you'll see, hear what you'll hear, and feel what you'll feel when it's going exactly the way you'd like it to). Run through this movie again and again in your mind (as if you're living it now) and feeling how good it feels in your body when it's going well.

A variation of this to use when goal setting is to imagine running through a movie of your life as it will be three years after you've achieved your goal (imagining you are living the life you'll have created for yourself). Watch this movie in your mind again and again, and notice what opportunities present themselves.

- **Change How You Feel Visualisation**

Another very simple way to change how you feel is simply to switch your attention to think of something that would bring a smile to your face – remembering a holiday, person, or good time. It's why many of us have photos all round the house – they remind us of people and times we want to remember. I'm sure you don't put up photos of what you'd like to forget!

4. L = Language.

This is what you think inwardly, what you say aloud, and what you write – about yourself, and anything in your outer word.

A common analogy for the mind is that of an iceberg – with the small tip above the water representing your conscious mind, and the much larger chunk of ice under the water representing your subconscious mind. There are various studies that quote differing views on the number of thoughts we have in a day – a commonly quoted figure is around 90,000, with only 10% of these being at a conscious level. While the majority (90%) of your thoughts being at a subconscious level.

Your subconscious mind stores all that has ever happened to you – your experiences, your memories, your thoughts, your feelings, emotional triggers, etc. You don't consciously tell your hand how to reach out and open a door. Nor do you tell your body to heal wounds, or your lungs to breathe – thankfully these all happen automatically. Conventional science usually says your mind stores information from the day you were born. However, there is growing evidence that this powerful recording machine is coding messages from when you were in your mother's womb and before you were conceived.

One of the reasons why it's so important to take control of your thoughts (at a conscious and subconscious level) is that, in the same way that the part underneath the water determines the direction of the iceberg, it's the powerhouse of your subconscious mind that drives your feelings and your actions. And thus, all the results you experience in life.

Your subconscious mind is thousands of times more powerful than your conscious mind. If you've ever consciously set yourself a goal but not achieved it, that's likely to have happened because you've had thoughts or emotional triggers in your subconscious mind which conflict with your conscious goal. Having contradictory stories running in your conscious and subconscious mind is a bit like having a little five-year-old boy on one end of the rope pulling as hard as he possibly can, with twenty strong, strapping twenty-five-year-old lads pulling the rope in the opposite direction. Who do you think is going win?

If you want to achieve success personally, in business, or at work, it's much easier to do so if all your thoughts and emotions are aligned to support you in achieving your goal.

And this is why in order to succeed in whichever way is important to you, it's vital to nurture positive thoughts and emotions. Any limiting beliefs or negative emotions will be hindering your success. When you align your conscious and subconscious mind, things will flow much easier.

But how do you do this if you aren't aware of the specific thoughts or emotional triggers that are holding you back, because they're in your subconscious mind? The wonderful resource you always have access to is your body, and specifically to the emotions you feel. These are an accurate projection of your subconscious programming. There are many different techniques you can use to re-programme your mind, and I'll share a couple of these shortly. But before I do, let's explore where your thoughts come from.

You've been shaped and moulded by everything you've experienced since you came into being in the womb and, before that, what the egg and sperm who united in your conception experienced in their evolution. From the moment you were born, people around you have told you what to think about yourself, about others, and about the world. As a young child, you were a sponge absorbing all you heard, saw and experienced. And because, until the age of six, children's brains have not evolved past the physical state of hypnosis ('theta' brain state),[40] what went on around you was being effectively recorded straight into your subconscious mind. You therefore quickly learned to believe others' opinions about you and where you fitted into society as being the truth, even though these were just others' thoughts and perspectives.

If you've been really lucky, you'll have heard lots of positive messages – such as 'I love you', 'you're wonderful', 'you're gorgeous', and other appropriate demonstrations of love. People may have encouraged you to do things, told you 'you can do it', supported you, and inspired you to embrace life to the full. However, you could have heard messages and experienced others' actions that led you to doubt yourself, dislike yourself, think you're not good enough, unworthy, or useless.

Few adults have taken the time to detox their subconscious mind of the beliefs they chose to take on as a child. Are you drifting through adulthood with thoughts about yourself which may be based on recordings you made of others, and which may not be true or serve you?

Today, you are effectively only the sum total of everything you've ever thought until now – about yourself, your potential, love, relationships, money, success, your work, business, or contribution to society. And spe-

40 Bruce Lipton, *The Biology Of Belief*, 2008, Hay House, p6

cifically, do you think it's possible for you to succeed? Do you think it's possible for you to be happy and successful doing what you love? Do you deserve to make it happen?

The good news is that in the same way that you've learned to believe today's truth, you can choose what you want to believe for the future. By replacing the beliefs and emotional triggers that hold you back with more resourceful programmes, you'll make it so much easier to succeed with confidence and ease.

Let me ask you this: have you ever had a hairstyle or an outfit that you loved, which you thought looked great and made you feel good at the time? But maybe now, when you look back at photos you think, 'what on earth was I doing?' Well, if you can change your mind about something that used to make you feel great, then you can also change the thoughts that are sabotaging your success!

How Do You Change Your Thoughts?

Whenever you learn something new, e.g. facts or a new skill, you are changing your thoughts. What I'm referring to here are the strategies you can use to change limiting beliefs you've got that no longer serve you. These broadly fall into these two categories:

1) those that you repeatedly practise consciously, e.g. affirmations and choosing positive language.
2) those that tackle the issue at a subconscious level, and which create instant and lasting change, e.g. tapping, NLP, hypnotherapy, Theta Healing, kinesiology, and many more interventions.

The main two I cover in this book are affirmations and tapping.

- **Affirmations**

This is the first way I learned to change my thoughts (and therefore my feelings, too), and in this context it's simply a positive statement. It works by consciously repeating positive statements to yourself several times a day until you've re-programmed your mind to unconsciously believe these new thoughts. To give you some ideas, I've listed affirmations at the end of chapters relating to the 9 Principles. And in Chapter 21, I share more about affirmations, including a brilliant model you can use to structure affirmations even when you don't know the underlying thoughts that are holding you back, or if you want to write affirmations to help you manifest your goals.

- **Tapping**

  I love tapping as it is really easy to learn; it can be used to overcome many things, including negative thoughts, emotions, trauma, pain, and cravings; it often makes you aware of the root cause of an issue so you can resolve this; it works quickly; has lasting impact (because it resolves issues at a subconscious level); and it works physically, mentally, and energetically. Tapping is the main technique we've been using with genocide survivors in Rwanda – because it is so effective in overcoming severe trauma. You can even use tapping to help manifest more money!

  Put simply, tapping is a bit like acupuncture without needles – by tapping on meridian energy points in the body, you neutralise negative emotions, pain, beliefs, and trauma.

  If you're familiar with tapping, I've listed suggested 'set up' statements at the end of each chapter which you may wish to use. I explain tapping more in Chapter 22.

5. E = Energy

I remember when I was growing up, I used to think my energy just came from what I ate and drank. But now I know there are so many other factors that influence our energy levels – what you spend your time doing; who you spend your time with; how you nurture your soul; how effectively you manage your emotions and take control of your thoughts; whether you are mindful or meditate; the quality of oxygen or air you are exposed to; how much sleep you get; your connection to nature and animals; and how much you exercise. All these things collectively have an impact on how you feel emotionally, physically, and energetically.

Many of the tools I've shared already will change your energy and energy vibration, including tapping, using your imagination, practising gratitude, and meditation. I also personally love how you can change how you feel by listening to music. I have playlists for running, chilling, reflecting, and working, and consciously select what I listen to so that I evoke the feeling I want in any situation. Essential oils and drinking home-made nutritious smoothies are another couple of my favourite daily energy boosters.

What boosts your energy?

How could you incorporate more of this into your daily life?

It may seem like a simple acronym but remembering to SMILE is a great way to change how you feel in the moment, particularly if you practise any of the techniques I've shared above.

Overcoming Negative Emotions

It's one thing to be able to change how you feel, but it's sometimes also healthy to experience negative emotions, e.g. experiencing grief, the loss of a loved one, or fear in extreme cases when it really is in your interest to fight for your survival. When your life is not at risk, it can be beneficial to allow yourself to experience the negative emotion so that you have greater insight and learning for the next time you're in a similar position. That said, it is appropriate to let go of these negative emotions once they have served their purpose. Here is a simple process you can follow to do this:

1. **Notice** – what you're feeling, consider why and what it could be beneficial for you to tackle.
2. **Release** – when it feels appropriate to let go of the negative feeling, e.g. using tapping.
3. **Replace** – do something that will make you feel better.

Sometimes going through this process may only take a few minutes; in the case of grief or trauma, it may take much longer and need the support of a practitioner. It's not good for you to hold onto negative emotions for too long, or to continually expose yourself to stress. And some emotions such as guilt don't serve you in a healthy way, other than to let you know there is something to forgive yourself.

Creating Lasting Change

Learning how to change how you feel in the moment, and realising you have this ability within you, can be liberating. But that's only part of the picture – if you keep taking headache tablets for your headaches but don't tackle the root cause, it will be an on-going saga.

One of the leaders in the development of Positive Psychology, Professor Martin Seligman, defines happiness as:

$$H = S + C + V$$

Where H is your enduring level of happiness (rather than short-term highs), S is your set range (or genetically coded 'happiness thermostat', C is the circumstances of your life, and V represents factors under your voluntary control.[41] In other words your happiness stems from a mixture of nature and nurture (how you were nurtured as a child and how YOU nurture yourself). Your genes and what happens to you in life are not the only factors that determine your happiness – a huge element of that's down to how you choose to manage your emotions.

One of the aspects that many therapeutic interventions miss is the value of positive experience and converting this into lasting change – so you feel good at a core level, and develop healthy habits that will support you in creating the life you want for yourself.

Neuropsychologist Rick Hanson, author of *Hardwiring Happiness*[42], has come up with a four-step HEAL process for doing this, which is very similar to many of the processes we use in NLP (Neuro-Linguistic Programming) & Hypnotherapy:

1. **Have** the positive experience (either noticing or creating the experience/feeling).
2. **Enrich** the experience, so you get lots of neurons in your brain to fire together and hardwire the new experience. You can do this by intensifying the experience; spending longer in the experience; bringing the experience down into your body; relating to what's new; noticing why this is important to you.
3. **Absorb** and turbo-charge the installation of this new way of being, e.g. by being fully present in the moment or visualising the positive experience entering your body.
4. **Link** this positive experience to the old negative thought/memory to neutralise the negative association.

In Summary

Rather than suffering upset, stress, feeling down, fear, anxiety or pain, recognise that negative emotions are your body's brilliant alarm system signalling that something's wrong and that it would like you to take remedial action. The SMILE model summarises the different type of tools you can use to do this.

So for example, if you are feeling anxious about the uncertainty that comes

41 *Martin E.P. Seligman, PHD, Authentic Happiness, 2002, Nicolas Brealey Publishing, p45*

42 *Hardwiring Happiness by Rick Hanson, published by Rider, 2013*

with working towards your goal, you could:

1. Smile.
2. Sit, stand, or walk about in the way you would if you were full of confidence and certainty.
3. Visualise yourself working confidently towards this, overcoming challenges, achieving your goal, and living a life as though you've already achieved it. Feel as though you've already achieved it.
4. Tell yourself – I can do this (doing tapping, if required, to overcome any anxiety you feel).
5. Do something that energises you and makes you feel good or raises your energy vibration.
6. Then to embed it all, keep doing what makes you feel good as you think about your goal, and notice what's different.
7. Repeat this process lots of times to hardwire your brain and body for success!

It really is so important that we all learn to manage our emotions – for our own health and that of those around us. We all have bad days and challenging times, but when you're feeling stressed, down, angry or hurt, do you really want your loved ones to feel the same way?

Resourceful Questions

- What triggers stress or anxiety for me?

- How could I let go of this?

- How could I discover which tools work best for me?

- What one thing could I do differently each day to create new healthy habits?

- How could I implement my ideas?

Empowering Affirmations

- I love smiling and bringing joy to others.

- It feels great to be able to let go of stresses.

- I love being able to change how I feel.

- I feel better each day.

- I deal with life's challenges with ease.

Tapping 'Set Up' Statements

- Even though I'm upset about XXX, I deeply and completely love and accept myself.

- Even though I'm not sure I believe I can easily change how I feel naturally, I'm willing to give it a shot.

- Even though I don't know why I feel this way, I deeply and completely love and accept myself.

Recommended Resources

- www.purehappiness.com

- *From Heartbreak To Happiness* by Kim Macleod

- *The Endorphin Effect* by William Bloom

- *Molecules Of Emotion AND Everything Your Need To Know To Feel Good* by Candace B. Pert

- *Feel The Fear And Do It Anyway* by Susan Jeffers

- *Creative Visualisation* by Shakti Gawain

- *Hardwiring Happiness* by Rick Hanson

- *It's The Thought That Counts* by Dr David R Hamilton

- *Authentic Happiness* by Martin E P Seligman

- www.authentichappiness.com - for lots of free on-line questionnaires and resources

- *Change Your Words Change Your World* by Andrea Gardner

Master How To Manage Your Emotions

I share several tools to help you learn how to manage your emotions on my website, including a short film on how to tap, a free relaxation audio, and other paid services – check out www.alisoun.com/heartatude.

Chapter 16

Principle 6 – Invite Possibility & Success

Open your mind and be curious about the endless possibilities for your success. Choose empowering thoughts and take inspired action to create opportunities and manifest your goals.

I remember hearing the adventurer Bear Grylls being interviewed on a radio show and being asked about what had been the catalyst for him living the unusual life he does – travelling the world doing many things which the rest of us think are mad. His response was that he had been brought up to believe that 'life is more interesting outside your comfort-zone'. Wow!

Just imagine being told as a young child that life could be more fun or interesting on the other side of your comfort zone! Do you think you'd have been more courageous? Could you have been more open to the possibility that it's okay to try something new? Or to dare to dream that your ideas were possible?

It's not who you are that holds you back, it's who you think you are.

Richard Branson is someone else who developed a very different approach to life's challenges than most of us, thanks in part to the trials he was set by his family when he was young. If you read his book *Screw It. Let's Do It*,[43] you'll get great insights into the mind of this visionary who comes up with many great ideas and solutions which push the realms of what the rest of us believe is possible.

Most people are capable of achieving far more than they believe is possible, but unfortunately their thoughts and feelings hold them back.

43 *Screw It Let's Do It, Lessons In Life by Richard Branson, Virgin Books, 2006*

Imagine how it would feel if every day you woke up believing it was possible to be the person you'd love to be; to achieve what you'd love to do; or to feel how you'd like to feel. Imagine believing that it is possible, that you have the ability to do it (or to learn how), and that you deserve to be happy and successful. Because you do!

One of the people interviewed in the film, 'The Secret', is a guy called Morris Goodman (or 'The Miracle Man', as he is better known). In March 1981, Morris was in a plane crash. His injuries were so severe that medical specialists thought that if he survived, he would remain in a vegetative state, completely paralysed, unable to breathe or eat without the support of machines. However, Morris refused to believe in that future for himself, and instead decided to use the only thing he was able to control – his mind – to mentally focus on how he wanted to recover physically. He went on to make a remarkable recovery and walked out of the hospital unaided a few months later (and within the timeframe he'd set for himself – Christmas that year).

What's Possible?

Your beliefs around whether something is possible or not are very dependent upon your life experiences and conditioning – often from what you've seen; or what you've heard or read to be true (from reputable sources). Collectively, these form parameters in our mind around the realms of possibility and success. And so, when you're presented with something you've either not experienced for yourself, or which conflicts with your current belief patterns, you may question whether it's possible – at all, and especially for you. A common approach is to automatically believe it's not possible unless proven otherwise.

But why is that? Why are many people's minds set to default to believe things are not true, don't work, are nonsense or impossible, until they have proof? Why don't they believe anything could be possible until proven otherwise?

It comes down to your conditioning – what you have been taught about possibility, and the 'need' for evidence.

What is your response when you're presented with a new idea or solution? Is it to explore how to make it happen or experience it for yourself? Or do you automatically dismiss new ideas, or get anxious when faced with a challenge that would take you outside of your comfort zone?

Have you ever achieved or learned how to do something that you once thought wouldn't be possible?

If you're of a certain age, you may remember the first time you heard about the Internet. I remember thinking the notion that people would sit in front of a monitor and – with the push of a button – be able to communicate with one another and even see each other on the screen, was far-fetched.

And as for mobile phones, they still blow my mind. How is it that if I tap a piece of glass or plastic, within a few seconds my text message manages to make its way around the world, through the information fog of invisible digital data, not only from the UK to Sydney but to find my friend's (no-one else's) mobile phone? And when she taps into her phone, I almost instantaneously get a reply? Sometimes I sit being mindful of what I'm doing when I'm texting, and I'm in awe at this incredible little gadget that's become an integral part of our lives. I still don't know HOW it works, but experience has taught me it does.

It's a bit like the ability for a jumbo jet to stay in the sky – it doesn't seem right to my mind (because I don't know how), but having seen for myself that they usually do, I know it's possible.

Are you someone who needs to know HOW? Or are you happy to 'evidence' things are possible, even if you don't know how? Just yesterday it was great to hear one of my friends share how she was a complete convert to homeopathic medicine – she'd always been a disbeliever until she'd tried it for herself and instantly been 'cured' of her ailments. Her mind-set had shifted from 'I don't get homeopathy' to 'it's amazing, you need to try it'.

Astonishing one-off events that challenge the realms of possibility are often called miracles, because we don't yet understand how something happened, or there is no immediate opportunity to replicate the situation to demonstrate it again, e.g. someone having the strength to lift a car off a child; someone recovering from an 'incurable' disease; or someone in sport smashing a previously held record, like the first time the mile was run in under four minutes by Roger Bannister. But over time, as technology advances and our understanding of science continues to evolve, some of what was previously considered miraculous becomes a new norm, e.g. IVF treatment giving many of those who haven't been able to conceive naturally the joy of having a family.

Until the 2012 Olympics in London, I believed that those who won medals had all been mastering their sport for many years and from a very early age. It certainly wasn't in my consciousness that anyone could take up a sport and win an Olympic medal in less than four years. But during these games, several in the UK team alone proved this was possible. And they inspired many of us to at least be open to the possibility that we could, too – even though many of us in our forties came to the conclusion that it's still highly unlikely, especially if we don't actually have the inclination to do so.

This brings me on to a really important point: I'm certainly not suggesting that *everything* is possible (as I know some people do). However, what I do encourage you to do is to give yourself permission to believe your dreams, and in your goals and aspirations. To trust that they could be possible – even if you don't yet know how. Be curious, explore the potential that they could happen, and trust that by taking steps towards your goal, the way forward will present itself. Don't give up just because you don't know how it will all work out.

It's a bit like driving along a country road in the dark with your headlights on – you can only see what's directly in front of you, but you trust your headlights will continue to show you the way until you reach your destination. And, while on your journey, you navigate your way around the bends, potholes, and any other challenges that you encounter along the way.

Developing a Success Mind-set

It's up to you to choose how you approach possibility and success – whether to believe something isn't possible because it doesn't 'fit' with your current way of thinking. Or, if you're up for an adventure, to see where the potential of success could take you.

When it comes to success and whether or not you succeed, it depends whether you have any doubts (consciously or unconsciously) that fall into these three different categories:

1. **Possibility** – whether or not you believe it's possible for <u>anyone</u> to achieve it.
2. **Ability** – whether you think <u>you</u> have the ability to do it.
3. **Worthiness** – whether you feel you deserve to succeed.

Possibility – in order to conceive that something is possible for you, you first need to believe that what you're aspiring to is possible at all (for anyone, including yourself). If you believe that it is impossible at this level, you're unlikely to believe that you'll master it. However, once you believe it's possible, you stand a much better chance.

Many of the inventions we rely upon in our daily lives today were invented by people who ignored their doubts and those of others. People like Thomas Edison (the light bulb); Alexander Graham Bell (the telephone); John Logie Baird (the TV); Sir Timothy John Berners-Lee (the Internet); and Alexander Fleming (Penicillin). They all persevered until their efforts paid off.

Have you ever tried fire-walking?

This was something I couldn't get my head around when I first heard of it, so I decided to go along to a seminar where this was one of the main activities. On a warm summer evening, I found myself marching along a bank of the River Thames in London with another 5,000 people, clapping, chanting, and moving to the sounds of African drums. In unison, we were all moving ever closer to the 40 or so fires that had been lit (each approximately 20 metres long). It was a surreal experience. We'd been reassured that if we followed the instructions we'd been given, we'd be fine as we walked across these hot coals with bare feet. That we'd receive no burns.

I had loads of doubts in my mind, but the people in front of me seemed to be managing fine, so I kept telling myself that if it was possible for them, it must be possible for me, too. When I got to the fire, I froze. But, led by the instructor, I raised my head and started to walk briskly but calmly over the coals saying, 'cold moss, cold moss, cold moss...' Once I'd crossed to the other side, I remember looking back and asking myself – did I really do that? How? I still didn't understand how, but now I did know it was possible. I'd just done what I'd previously thought wasn't possible and that I'd been terrified to try. It was so liberating!

The next day I remember speaking to a guy who hadn't been quite so blown away by the experience, as he'd been brought up in a country where they walked through much bigger fires from a young age. For as long as he could remember, fire-walking was something he thought everyone did. What a great example of the differences in cultural conditioning!

Ability – once you believe that something is possible, the next level of doubt you could encounter relates to whether or not you think you have the ability to do it. Have you ever said to yourself, or aloud – 'I can't'? When you do, this is an indication that you are stuck at an ability level – you accept it's possible, or that others can do it, but you haven't yet mastered how to do it yourself.

Often when we say 'I can't', it's a habitual response that has other deeper meaning such as 'I don't know how to – yet'. The problem is that when you interpret 'I can't' as being the 'truth', it holds you back from achieving your goals. A more effective strategy is to instead treat these times of doubt as learning opportunities, as summed up in the popular statement – *'there is no such thing as failure, only feedback'.*

When Thomas Edison was trying to get the prototypes for the 'light bulb' to work, people around him were questioning what he was doing, because in their minds what he was doing wasn't working (and would never work). But his perception was that he was eliminating what wouldn't work until he worked out what actually did.

Thankfully, most of us are not involved in life or death situations, or decisions every day where we could kill someone. So choosing to believe we have 'failed' in a way that is permanent or 'bad' is not helpful. Nor does it nourish your soul.

However, if you choose to learn from situations where you don't get the result you were hoping for, and then refine your next attempt, you'll be far more likely to achieve your goal. And in doing so, you will expand your comfort zone, what you believe about success, and boost your resilience.

We live in a fast-paced world where we've become conditioned to get instant or quick results – instant coffee, ready-made meals, next day deliveries, etc. And so many people set themselves up for disappointment when they expect to get great results the first time they try something new.

Often, after a popular talent show or sporting event has been aired, there is a surge of people who have been inspired to learn to sing or take up a new sport. Some think about it for a few days but take no action. Others take it as far as joining a course to learn how to master this new talent. Of those who attend the first class, there will be people who will think after one attempt that they 'can't do it' or are 'useless', so they decide not to go back to the class. They have compared their initial efforts to the people they've seen on TV who have been honing their skills for years! Some people will go back to the second class, but gradually those continuing will drop off week by week as more of them question whether or not they can do it – because they are not recognising the effort it takes to learn a new skill.

Yet they did when they learned to walk. There will have been a time when you couldn't walk, but you were observing most people around you walking, so you didn't doubt that one day you could do it, too. But before you could walk, you would have tried many times to pull yourself up while holding onto furniture or someone's legs, before falling down. And each time you fell down, you may have had a pause, but then you got up and tried again. And again. And again. Until you developed the physical strength in your legs and body that enabled you to walk.

Now, just imagine if as an adult you applied the same approach to everything you'd love to achieve in life. That if, when you give things a shot and you don't get the results you want, you accept this is part of your learning experience. That you treat each attempt as an opportunity to get feedback on how you can refine your approach, and keep trying until you succeed.

'The greatest glory in living lies not in never falling, but in rising every time we fall.'

Nelson Mandela

Worthiness – when you believe that it's possible for you to learn to succeed at doing something, you are far more likely to do it. Although this third level of limiting beliefs, relating to whether or not you believe and feel you deserve to succeed, could still sabotage your success.

As I've said earlier in this book, each and every one of us was born into this world with exactly the same rights in terms of our self-worth and our rights to be loved, respected, happy, and to succeed. But through the course of growing up, the way you have interpreted what you've been exposed to could have led you to question these universal rights. Do you ever think or feel:

• I'm not good enough to. . ?

• My opinions/ideas are not worth listening to?

• I don't deserve to. . ? Relating to a positive outcome, e.g. to succeed or be happy.

• I deserve to. . ? Relating to a negative outcome, e.g. to fail or be unhappy.

• I'm not worth. . ?

If you do, then these thoughts and feelings will be hindering your success, to some extent. Remember, your life today is a manifestation of all the thoughts you've had until today. If you change those that no longer serve you, you'll be surprised at how easy it is to start getting better results.

Not only is it possible for you to achieve far more than you currently think you are capable of – you also deserve to succeed!

Embarking Upon Your 'Hero's Journey'

In her wonderful book *The Wizard Of Us*,[44] Jean Houston explains Joseph Campbell's 7-step Hero's Journey that is often used as an effective structure for making good movies. It also gives great insight into the process you may go through when you have a calling or desire for change:

1. **Call to adventure** – your desire to leave the old and venture into the new.
2. **Refusal of the call** – giving in to doubts until you can no longer resist moving forward.
3. **Guardian of the threshold** – experiencing an unfriendly being(s) who prefers the old way or status quo, e.g. Cinderella's wicked stepmother.
4. **The belly of the whale** – the lowest point of your journey as you take steps into the unknown and embrace the potential of a new world.
5. **Road of trials** – the time when you will be tested until you find the resources to keep you going and survive (often the fighting scenes in the movie).
6. **Meeting with the beloved** – recognition from someone important, and potential reward (e.g. the Philosopher's stone).
7. **Master of two worlds** – when you consolidate your new experiences with the old world, to create a new world going forward.

I just love this model, and I've found it especially reassuring to realise that as I venture into new arenas, feeling nervous or challenged by others is just part of the natural process of change on my journey.

How to Enjoy More Possibility & Success

In the last chapter I talked about the power of two techniques – affirmations and tapping (with further details in chapters 21 and 22). Below you'll find some resourceful questions, affirmations, and tapping statements, to help you come up with exciting goals and overcome any doubts, anxieties, worries or insecurities about achieving these.

---

44. *The Wizard of Us: Transformational Lessons From Oz by Jean Houston, Beyond Words Publishing,* 2012

Another great way to accelerate your success is to speak to and learn from those who know how to do what you love – whether it's to have a chat, ask them questions, attend one of their events, read their books, or watch their YouTube channel.

In Summary

There are many people in the world who have achieved remarkable things against the odds, and you can, too, if you put your mind to it. Whatever you aspire to achieve or be, you are far more likely to succeed if you choose to believe (at a conscious and subconscious level) that it's possible, that you have the ability to make it happen, and that you deserve to succeed! Because you do… it's simply a case of connecting to what is important to you, or makes your heart sing; deciding what specifically you'd love to achieve; and doing what it takes to overcome any obstacles along your journey.

Resourceful Questions

• If xxx was possible, what would I do?

• If I could do xxx, what would I do?

• How could I learn to xxx?

• How could I make this happen?

• Who could help me achieve this?

Affirmations

• It's possible, I can do it, I deserve it.

• It's possible for me to XXX.

• I have the ability to XXX.

• I deserve to XXX.

• I love learning how to make things happen.

• I make things happen and get great results.

Tapping 'Set Up' Statements

• Even though I don't have a clue how I'll do this, I deeply and completely love and accept myself.

• Even though I'm not sure this is really possible, I'm open to the possibility that it is.

- Even though I may make mistakes along the way, I'm OK with that.

Recommended Resources

- *The Wizard Of Us* by Jean Houston

- *Awaken The Giant Within* by Anthony Robbins

Chapter 17

Principle 7 – Act Consciously With Positive Intention

Consciously choose the focus of your attention, define your desired outcomes and consider positive intentions ahead of responding to people/situations, and then consciously take action aligned to these.

As human beings we spend most of our time operating on autopilot without conscious thought or intervention.

To some extent it needs to be this way so that the many miraculous activities of your body function and keep you alive. Thankfully, we don't need to remember to tell our heart to beat or our lungs to breathe – it just happens.

However, unconscious beliefs, habits, and emotional triggers can result in undesirable feelings and outcomes that conflict with what you'd like at a conscious level. Particularly at times when you feel challenged, as your subconscious mind takes over to 'protect' you from danger.

Remember, you have around 90,000 thoughts a day with most of these at a subconscious level. So unless you've done a thorough detox of your mind, the chances are that you are currently acting and making decisions based on out-dated subconscious habitual beliefs and programming that you no longer serves you. Beliefs and emotional triggers that will be making it harder than it needs be for you to achieve your goals or to be able to.

Plus, your mind can only cope with a fraction of the new information it is presented with each day. And so it disregards what it doesn't perceive as important, to prevent it going into overwhelm. That's fine if it's choosing to ignore information that isn't of interest or relevant to you. But how does your subconscious mind know what to look out for, unless you give it conscious nudges?

Many misunderstandings and upsets are caused by people acting without thinking. A lack of conscious thought often contributes to time and money being wasted, poor decisions being made, relationships breaking down, people going into debt, the nurturing of addictions and bad habits that result in unnecessary illness. And sadly in extreme cases, being disconnected to our hearts and acting unconsciously from a place of fear or scarcity can escalate into conflict, disputes, and even wars – with terrible consequences for so many people. Sometimes even when we're well intended, our unconscious programming can cause us to act in a way that results in others suffering unnecessary stress, upset or anxiety.

I'll never forget one early morning flight from Edinburgh Airport. As someone who used to be an anxious flier, over the years I've learned to calm my nerves and now quite enjoy it – unless there is increased reason to feel concerned. On a lovely clear and calm morning, the plane appeared to shudder and make more noise than normal during take-off. But thankfully, the cabin crew seemed to be going about their usual routine, and all seemed well. Or at least that was what I thought until the pilot came over the tannoy and apologised for the bumpy take-off. If he'd stopped there, it would have been fine, but as he went on to let us know this had been due to problems with the undercarriage, you could feel the anxiety in the cabin rise. Particularly after we were told the emergency services would be greeting us on the runway when we landed.

I'd like to think his intentions were good, that he intended to reassure us all was well. But for quite a few of us on the flight, he'd given us too much information. We now had an hour or so to worry about whether we'd land safety. Had it not been so early in the morning, I may have wondered if the pilot was on commission for alcohol sales on the flight!

Turning Off Your Auto-pilot

Acting consciously with positive intention is about switching off your autopilot – so you are more present in the moment and consciously make decisions aligned to what you'd like or love to achieve. Then acting from your heart and taking action towards your desired outcome(s) whilst at the same time being unattached to these. Letting go of any ego; knowing that you do the best you can in any given moment, and trusting the laws of the Universe to manifest whatever is in your highest interest.

'Insanity is repeating the same mistakes and expecting different results.'

Narcotics Anonymous

Obviously, for the situations where you are already getting the results that you want, there is no need to do anything different. However, applying this principle is really helpful in situations where what you're doing isn't working, when you're doing something new or important, or when you are feeling challenged. It is a great strategy for boosting your performance and getting better results in all areas of life.

The Scope of Intention

In his book *The Power of Intention*, Dr Wayne Dyer shares a couple of different ways to interpret 'intention':

• At one end of the spectrum it's 'a strong purpose or aim accompanied by the determination to produce a desired result'.[45] Based on the existence of free will, that you can consciously choose to think, feel and act in a way that's aligned to a specific result that you'd like to achieve.

• While it's also a force that exists in nature. The energy field that we're all part of, that's within us, and which guides us towards our destiny – without any conscious thought, e.g. spring turns to summer, babies grow to become adults. The premise that what's meant for you won't go past you – whether you articulate this as karma, fate, or your soul's purpose. And even the possibility that this unconscious intention may influence the scope of our free will.

In her books *The Field* and *The Intention Experiment*, Lynne McTaggart offers another dimension. She shares copious examples of scientific studies by well-respected scientific institutions that suggest 'human thoughts and intentions are an actual physical "something" with the astonishing power to change our world. Every thought we have is a tangible energy with the power to transform'.[46] So whether your thoughts are positive or negative, they could be shaping the reality of not only how you feel, but also having an effect on what manifests in your outer world.

In the context of this principle, the emphasis is on setting conscious

---

45   *The Power Of Intention, Dr Wayne W Dyer, Hay House, 2004, p3.*

46 *The Intention Experiment, Use Your Thoughts To Change The World, Lynne McTaggart, HarperElement, 2008, p7.*

intentions while accepting there is also a greater energy force at play. I like refining my focus by considering two different aspects of intention: the outcomes you'd like to happen; and the part you play in achieving these outcomes (i.e. how you intend to be, and what you intend to do to achieve these outcomes).

Recently I was surprised to hear one of my friends talking about how she found it really easy to float on her back in the sea – not just for a few seconds, but effortlessly floating for quite a few minutes at a time. Swimming has never been something I've found easy – I've always had to put a lot of effort into not sinking. However, my friend had a completely different perspective and it was fascinating to hear how from a young age she'd been taught that the water would support her – that as human beings we can naturally float. This was a completely new concept to me and certainly hadn't been my experience. But was that because I was focusing on not sinking rather than floating? And because I believed my default was to sink, rather than to float?

The next time I went swimming, I consciously decided to visualise gliding along the top of the water and to hold the belief that the water would hold me up. And I was stunned at how much easier it was! My desired outcome was the same – to swim effortlessly. However, by consciously shifting my attention (to override habitual thinking) and choosing to engage with this activity differently, I at last enjoyed the previously elusive outcome I'd yearned for.

The 5-Steps to Taking Conscious Action

If you, too, want to boost the results that you're getting, this process will help you do this. Especially if it's applied ahead of doing something for the first time; mastering a new skill; doing something where the outcome is really important to you; dealing with a challenging situation or person; to turnaround a negative situation: or where other strategies haven't worked.

1. Stop and become fully present in the moment

Becoming more aware of the present moment first involves consciously deciding to stop doing what you were about to do. To stop, take a few deep breaths, and connect to your heart before taking any further action.

Sometimes this may involve turning off the internal chatterbox in your mind that distracts you from the present moment, with superfluous thoughts about the past and the future. Or it may be more appropriate to manage your emotions and to put yourself in a good emotional state. You can get ideas for how to do this in Chapters 11 and 15.

> *'The mind is a superb instrument if used rightly.*
> *Used wrongly, however, it becomes very destructive.'*
> **Eckhart Tolle**

To develop the ability to experience being fully present, many people start by learning how to quieten their mind, e.g. through meditation. Whatever technique you decide to use, you could set aside time each day to do this.

Or you could apply this 5-step process to a situation you regularly find challenging in advance, so you are better prepared in the moment.

2. Define your desired outcomes

One of the great disciplines I learned from training in NLP is to focus on your desired outcomes ahead of taking any action. To focus on the positive and what you'd like to happen rather than what you don't want. This could relate to long-term goals or activities in the immediate future.

Do you ever think or talk about what you don't want rather than defining what you do want?

I am still pleasantly surprised at how consciously considering my desired outcomes, before taking any action, yields so much more clarity, focus, and direction. Just doing this one thing helps me make better decisions about what to do, what to say, and/or how to be. And I've found asking others to do the same when they are stuck or dealing with a challenging situation, is a great help to them, too.

Where the outcome you're working towards involves others, it's also worth considering the potential desired outcomes of the other person, so you are also mindful and compassionate in your interactions.

3. Choose how you intend to be and FEEL it!

This relates to the part you commit to play in creating your desired outcomes. How you intend to be and what you intend to do, e.g. to be positive rather than negative; to be confident rather than giving in to nerves; to respond calmly to challenges; to be open-minded; to try new things; and to open your heart and embrace all the heart values (love, kindness, compassion, respect, peace, gratitude or integrity).

4. Take action aligned to your desired outcomes

In terms of what you do and how you act. Remembering to put yourself into an appropriate positive emotional state first. You could do this by visualising things going the way you'd like them to go – all the way through to the point you've experienced your desired outcomes (and overcome challenges you may face). By tapping or using any of the techniques you find most effective.

5. Be unattached to your goals or desired outcomes

An important aspect of attracting the outcomes you'd like is to let go of any attachment to them. What I mean by this is that while you'd love to achieve your desired outcomes, your future happiness or worthiness is not dependent upon attaining them. That once you've defined your desired outcomes, you accept you will do your best and trust the Universe to manifest whatever is in your highest good. To feel this trust in your heart, that whatever happens in the future is the perfect solution, even if it doesn't feel it at the time.

Because when we're attached to outcomes, we've usually stepped into our ego or are acting from a place of scarcity or fear rather than love or peace in our hearts. This in turn can lead to feelings of disappointment, frustration, upset, anger, or a lack of worthiness, if things don't work out in the way we hope.

And sometimes there is something else at play – it could be that you've set goals you don't have enough control or influence over. Or you may have conflicting subconscious beliefs or feelings that mean your personal energy vibration isn't aligned to what you say you want. And also remember your personal brand (the way you are perceived by others) also impacts the results that you get. It could even be fate, karma, or that your soul purpose is that you experience something different.

So whenever you set yourself a goal or desired outcome, notice what you feel about achieving it. And manage your emotions so that you feel peace rather than any unhealthy and unproductive feelings.

I remember working beside someone who used to push an emotional trigger inside me whenever she was around. It was one of those situations where we didn't particularly like each other, but needed to learn to get on in order to do the jobs we were paid to do. And so, ahead of meetings with her I'd go into a meeting room for a few minutes and do a number of things: I'd use affirmations to lessen any anxiety or frustration I was feeling (I didn't know tapping at that point); then I'd get clear on the desired outcomes I wanted to achieve from our meeting; and how I intended to be e.g. calm, positive and honest (even if this took a lot of conscious effort). Doing this didn't change the fact that I wouldn't have chosen to be in her company, but choosing to change how I interacted with her certainly helped me build a more functional working relationship with her.

It's OK to Get it Wrong Sometimes

Have you ever:

• planned to do something and acted differently in the moment?

• impulsively done something you later regret?

• or done what you intended to do with positive intention but others interpreted what you did differently?

The reality is that every time you interact with others they will always interpret your message differently to the way you intended. We've all been through our own unique life experience and therefore the unconscious filters we process information through in our minds, will draw different conclusions. The art of a good communicator is someone who effectively closes the gap between intended and interpreted messages.

Sometimes it can also be hard to know what the best thing to do – both in advance and in the moment. Hindsight can be helpful if we acknowledge it from the perspective of learning how we could handle a similar situation better in the future. But not if we are critical or beat ourselves up.

It breaks my heart when travelling in places of great poverty, with kids running around the streets with no shoes, or the child beggars on the streets of India (many of whom have had limbs cut off by cruel 'benefactors' so they fetch more money). When you see the desperate pleas for survival in their eyes as they hold out a hand to you, what is the right thing to do? If you give one kid money, hundreds will descend upon you in a matter of seconds. Is giving them money really helping them? Or lining the pockets of those they are 'working' for? We can't solve everyone's problems and so the approach I adopt is to focus on helping those I can.

In whatever situation you're in, you can only do your best in that moment. Remember the most you can control (or learn to manage) is what you think, what you feel, and what you do in response to that external event. Choosing to switch off your autopilot, and taking the time to align your thoughts and feelings to your desired outcomes, will get you better results. You'll have more conscious awareness of things to celebrate. And if you choose to reflect and learn from what doesn't work, you'll have ideas for what to do differently in the future.

Defusing Others' Negative Behaviours With Intention

I used to have someone in my life that sometimes came across as mean and unkind. They often put other people down, as though doing this and making others feel bad, helped them to feel good. I'd noticed them doing this to others for a while before they made the mistake of adopting the same approach with me. You see, rather than giving in to their demands or 'fighting' back (as others tended to do) I simply said, 'I'm confused, what's the intention behind what you've just said?'

Watching their reaction to my response was like watching a cartoon character being hit over the head with a mallet – as though stars had appeared above them and their eyes were spinning round and round. There was a look of confusion on their face before they turned their back on me and walked away.

I obviously don't know what was going through their minds as they took in what I'd said. But my response certainly stopped them in their tracks. Which makes me wonder whether they realised their intention towards me wasn't a good one, and didn't want to admit this about themselves. I didn't really care; all I knew was that this one simple question asked calmly and with peace in my heart, defused a situation that could have been confrontational. And they never attempted their bullying tactics on me again.

Asking others to clarify their intentions in this way works in all sorts of situations – the secret is to make sure you come from a place of love, kindness, and compassion (and display congruent language, tonality, and body language) when doing this.

In Summary

If you'd like to experience something better or different in any area of your life, acting consciously with positive intention is one of the easiest principles to master and will make a huge difference. Applying this will help you feel better, make smarter decisions, get better results, and feel more in control of your destiny.

Resourceful Questions

These are three of the most powerful questions that you can ask yourself ahead of taking any action:

• What is my desired outcome?

• How do I intend to be?

• What do I commit to do to achieve this?

Empowering Affirmations

• I intend to be positive and calm even when I am challenged.

• I intend to listen and be open-minded.

• I intend to ask questions.

Tapping 'Set Up' Statements

• Even though I don't always get it right, I deeply and completely accept I always do the best I can.

• Even though I don't always get the results I'd like, I deeply and completely love and accept myself.

• Even though I sometimes speak without thinking, I deeply and completely love and accept myself.

Recommended Resources

• *The Power Of Intention* by Wayne Dyer

• *The Seven Laws Of Success* by Deepak Chopra

• *The Intention Experiment* & *The Field* by Lynn McTaggart

• *The Power Of Now* by Eckhart Toll

Chapter 18

Principle 8 – Develop Meaningful Connections & Relationships

Reconnect with the inner essence of who you really are. Make time to relate and connect with others, to be truly present in their company, and to build harmonious and fruitful relationships with all you interact with.

Your ability to be happy, healthy, and successful is very much dependent upon the connections and relationships you nurture. The relationships you have with yourself, others, nature, the planet, what you consume, with money, and how you approach success.

• How do you invest time and energy building good relationships?

• Do you feel energized or drained by your current relationships?

• Do your relationships with money, food, drink or exercise support or hinder your success?

Life is a lot easier when you surround yourself with people who love you, who support you and genuinely want the best for you. By contrast, you can make it a lot harder for yourself by spending time with those who only offer you love on their terms, who put you down, who rubbish your ideas or opinions, and are more interested in encouraging you to do what's best for them.

What you feel about yourself impacts all areas of your life and particularly the quality of the relationships you attract. These in turn influence the opportunities that present themselves and therefore shape your success.

The relationships you had as a child with each of your parents (or primary care-givers) have a huge impact on how you feel about yourself and where you 'fit' in the world.

If you were lucky enough to have enjoyed lots of love, support, and encouraging attention when you were young, you're likely to have a better perspective of what a healthy relationship is than someone who is still suffering the emotional wounds of indifference, absence, neglect or abuse. If you didn't experience unconditional love when young, the good news is that in most situations it is possible to heal yourself so you can enjoy happy and healthy relationships in adulthood.

The people you attract into your life at any given time are often a direct reflection of the way you're thinking and feeling at that time. When you embrace the 9 Principles Of Heart-Centered Success, you're more likely to attract and enjoy fruitful relationships – because you'll be strong enough emotionally to avoid or let go of damaging relationships.

During my most recent trip to Rwanda, we asked our young team what's changed since joining our programme. They are all still living 'below the poverty line' by Western standards, but this was barely mentioned. What they all talked about was having gone from feeling helpless about the future to now having faith and optimism about what it holds. And the main contributing factors they mentioned were the connections and relationships they now have:

• How they feel about themselves – they've learned to love themselves wholeheartedly and to feel that they deserve to be loved, to be happy, and to succeed, in a way they didn't before.

• The love, support, and acceptance they have from one another – some have gone from having no other living relatives to now feeling part of a unique new family; one that's in constant contact regularly, gets together, and where everyone looks out for each other. They feel they have an emotional safety net now.

• The connections and relationships they have in a wider community – their sense of self-worth has undoubtedly been boosted by the support of international sponsors, their acceptance at university, or as leaders in their communities. And because they are now also helping those impacted by the Sandy Hook Elementary School massacre in the US, to overcome their grief.

Life in Rwanda may be far removed from your life, but I'll bet you've got similar needs to these young people – to love and to feel loved; to feel good about yourself; to feel happy; to be accepted; to feel safe; to laugh and have fun with other like-minded souls; to bring joy to others; and to succeed.

Relationships are the glue that support us through life and give us a sense of belonging – in families, communities, and cultures. We are hard-wired to be social; our need for social interaction as human beings is one of many reasons why as a species we've evolved and our global population has grown to over seven billion (more than double that of 1960).[47]

As you read through this chapter, I invite you to reflect on the types of relationship you are experiencing in your life right now and to consider if there are any changes you'd like to make. Being mindful of the fact that in order to change your relationships, this first involves changing yourself and how you interact with others.

The relationships (beliefs and feelings) you have in relation to all other aspects of life, such as your family, money, success, health, education, nutrition, work, religion or your community, also influence your success. As does the extent to which you are connected to your heart (principle one), your soul's path or your truth, and the beautiful person you were born to be. Unhealthy social conditioning creates disconnection and negative or destructive relationships. Which again highlights the importance of taking control of your mind and emotions so you give yourself the best chance of success.

The State of Healthy Relationships

This principle is about developing positive relationships that will support, nourish, and help you to enjoy your best life.

When you have a good relationship with yourself, you engage your heart in the way you treat yourself and feel good about who you are. A healthy, harmonious relationship with others is one where you have nurtured the ability to operate independently as an adult, while at the same time enjoy being part of a mutually beneficial partnership – one of interdependence, where each party thrives despite their differences, each are treated with love, kindness, compassion, integrity, respect, gratitude, and peace. Where there is a healthy balance of give and take. When you make time for one another and are truly present in each other's company. In other words, creating times when you give others your undivided attention – e.g. being fully present and attentive with them; listening more than you are talking; turning off your TV or mobile phone; putting down your computer or book, etc.

---

47 *United Nations, 1999, The World at Six Billion Report, p5.*

'Meaningful relationships cannot exist where there are two independent parties. It is our nature to be interdependent beings in relationship with one another.'

Lynn Serafinn, Author

However, in some relationships, the balance of interdependence has been lost or has never existed. This is where there is a lack of connection and you may get one or both parties acting completely independently of each another. Such relationships rarely bring out the best in either party, and are not usually sustainable in the long-term.

Of course, as we navigate our way through the trials of life, even the healthiest of relationships may lose that balance of interdependence from time to time. And that's OK. Sometimes we do 'need' more love and support from one another to get through life's challenges. However, when this happens, if you want to feel better and recapture a healthy relationship again, it's vital to recognise when it's time to proactively pick yourself up (and get support to help you do this if necessary), or to encourage this in the other person.

Some people don't know how to put themselves in a good emotional place, and struggle to get their needs met. When this happens, they may become desperately unhappy, stressed, overly dependent on others, or adopt unhealthy coping strategies, e.g. overeating, drinking excessively, taking drugs, going out on a spending spree or participating in other forms of escapism. Some revert into behaving or acting as a child rather than as an adult, and may be perceived as being 'needy' by those around them. One party not taking any responsibility for themselves (e.g. not getting the help they need when there is scope for them to do so) is not a healthy or sustainable situation for either party – particularly if either party wants to be happy.

Looking after someone with emotional challenges in the short-term is a kind and loving thing to do. However, sometimes doing so in adult relationships over the long-term can feed an over-dependence upon you. You may become a co-dependent, helping to keep them reliant on you rather than helping them be happy and self-sufficient. In such situations the hardest yet kindest thing may be to step back from the relationship (temporarily or permanently), or to get them professional support so they learn how to fend for themselves again – particularly if their behaviours are having a negative impact on the lives of others. Just because they 'need' love and support, doesn't mean you are the best person to provide it.

Developing healthy relationships with different aspects of your life is also important, e.g. how you think, feel and act around money, food, drink, exercise. Do your beliefs nurture a positive relationship that supports you in your quest for happiness and success? Or are any of these an unhealthy way to get a personal need met (e.g. to feel good in the moment)?

The relationships you experience, with people or other areas of your life, are all connected with what you think and feel about yourself, as well as being intricately linked to one another.

Your Relationship With Yourself

The most important relationship to develop first is what you think and feel about yourself.

If you want others to love you, the first secret is to love yourself. If you want others to be kind to you, be kind to yourself first. If you'd like others to help you – make helping yourself as well as others one of your mottos. If you'd like to live an authentic happy life, you first need to know who you are and what brings you joy. When you treat yourself well, you'll find most around you will treat you well, too. However, if you mistreat yourself (e.g. being negative, self-critical, doubtful, or letting others abuse or bully you), you're more likely to find that you attract those who will oppress you.

So many people drift through life disconnected from the unique and beautiful pure essence of who they are – they've lost sight of their natural self that's become hidden inside. Instead, they define themselves with labels, e.g. what they do, what they have, or who they know. These may be aspects of themselves, but they are not the unique spirit at the core of who they are. It can be a real balancing act remaining true to yourself while taking on different roles in life, but it is possible. And the starting point is to work out what you can control and influence, then engage your heart, and take action towards being the best person you were born to be, embracing possibility and success, and managing your emotions.

When you step into loving yourself and being authentic in all you do, opportunities to develop brilliant relationships will present themselves.

Enjoy Harmonious Relationships With Others

As human beings, most of us have the need to be loved and accepted – we are social animals by nature and so it's normal to form relationships and friendships with those we relate to. However, not all relationships are good – you can proactively choose to engage in positive healthy relationships, or you can allow yourself to be pulled into someone else's agenda.

'I've learned that people will forget what you said, people will forget what you did, but people will never forget how you made them feel.'

Maya Angelou, Author

Very few people succeed by themselves. To some extent their success is dependent upon the connections they make and the relationships they invest in. While there are times in our lives when we may feel we 'need' to be in relationships with those we wouldn't choose (e.g. at school or at work), most adults have more freedom to choose which relationships to cultivate and cherish, versus those it would be best to say 'no' to.

When you decide to make a change or explore something new in your life, one of the best ways to make this easier and more enjoyable is to build relationships with others who are already doing well in a similar situation. So you can share ideas and support one another.

Remember, how you feel is influenced by the emotional state of others around you, and so it's critical that you not only learn to manage your own emotions but also that you make smart choices about those you spend time with. The relationships you participate in with others determine the situations you experience – do you want these to be opportunities aligned to your dreams, or for your relationships with these people to hold you back?

I remember a few years ago a potential colleague at work was offered a job in our team. However, before she decided whether to accept the job, she first asked whether she could meet the team. At the time, we (the team she would join) thought this rather odd. But I now look back on this as such a good idea – if you're going to spend the majority of your waking time around others, making sure you connect with them is a great idea. I can't imagine myself now working with colleagues I don't relate to. It also showed great self-assurance on her part.

• What type of relationships do you have with your family and friends?

• What type of personal relationships have you experienced?

- What type of relationships do you have with colleagues or business associates?

- What part have you played in creating these relationships?

I feel very blessed to have good relationships with so many wonderful people – many lead similar lives to me, while others have very different experiences, interests and opinions. But everyone in my life has similar core values, and at some point we forged a special connection that I hope will remain with us for the rest of our lives.

We're all on a different journey through life and so it's natural to drift apart from some people. While I was initially a reluctant user of social media, I must admit that I now love feeling more connected to people I'm sure I would have lost touch with before now – not through any conscious act, but merely because life has taken us in different directions and there is only so much time in a day.

'If civilization is to survive, we must cultivate the science of human relationships – the ability of all peoples, of all kinds, to live together, in the same world at peace.'[48]

Franklin D. Roosevelt, US President

It's healthy to choose who you'd like to spend your time with, e.g. in terms of the values, qualities, and interests or common experiences with people you'd like to have in your life. And to say 'no' to people who ask to connect or meet up, if you don't want to nurture a relationship with them.

If you surround yourself with people who love and support who you are, you're more likely to be happy, try new things, and overcome life's challenges. However, if you choose to be in relationships with those who mock you, put you down or mistreat you, you'll have a very different experience of life.

You deserve to be happy, to be loved, to be respected, to be treated well in all your relationships. Sometimes the thought of initiating change or leaving a dysfunctional relationship may feel scary, but there are people who can support you and help you to work out the best way forward for you – this could be professionals or others who have overcome similar challenges.

Being in any type of relationship involves commitment and effort on your part. I know some people who claim they are unhappy with certain

---

48 *http://www.brainyquote.com/quotes/topics/topic_relationship2.html#54iGYrTbjxVPTVxy.99*

relationships in their life and yet don't prioritise the other person or are unpleasant to them. And they wonder why that person isn't keen to spend time with them! Everyone has the right to choose who to spend time with. Most of us juggle spending time with those who are most important to us – those we love, who we connect with, who we can have fun with, and who nourish our soul.

The first step to developing good relationships is to consider all your existing relationships and to decide how you could make a better contribution to the relationship. Here are a few ways to make a huge difference to the quality of conversations and relationships:

- We all have a natural communication style, e.g. introvert versus extrovert, focused on people versus tasks, loud or softly spoken, those who drill into detail versus those who focus on the big picture. Many conflicts are caused by people having different communication styles, and simply learning to understand your own natural style relative to others can help build more harmonious relationships. There are many resources for doing this, including a system I use with clients called DISC Behavioural Profiles.

- A basic need in most of us is to feel valued, worthy, and listened to. And yet so many people text, take non-critical calls, or do something else while 'listening' to others'. Giving others your undivided attention and actively listening to them enhances all relationships.

- Rather than jumping in with your story or opinions, remain silent or ask questions to enable the other person to fully express their perspective or ask how you can help – you have two ears and one mouth for a reason.

For relationships you no longer wish to remain part of, decide how you'll communicate this to the other party – this could be to let the relationship naturally drift apart, or may involve taking specific action, depending upon the nature of the relationship. Please remember to get the necessary support and guidance before making any life-changing decisions.

Your Relationship With Other Aspects Of Life

Your relationship with money

This is a huge and important topic – especially if you've set yourself financial goals or goals that need money.

Having delivered several workshops on developing the mind-set for financial abundance, it never ceases to amaze me how participants experience unexpected windfalls when they let go of negative thoughts, feelings, and energy around money.

I usually start these courses off by asking participants to complete the following statements:

• Money……..

• I…….. money

• Rich people are……

Obviously, if you think that money is bad, that rich people are mean, or you hate money, these beliefs will be sabotaging your financial success – because your subconscious mind will do everything within its power for you not to be 'bad' or 'mean'. Thinking or feeling you <u>need</u> to have money to be happy or successful carries a negative emotional charge that will cause all sorts of problems, e.g. neglecting your family or health when working long hours in pursuit of money.

Money is neither good nor bad – it's simply a form of energy exchange. It's what people do with it or do to get it that is sometimes questionable. The notion that 'money doesn't bring you happiness' is based upon the fact that you don't need money to be happy, and that some people with money are unhappy. However, for some reason many people have interpreted this statement as needing to choose between money and happiness. That you can't be happy and have money – what madness! That's like saying you can only have a right or a left arm, but not both. While money doesn't always bring happiness, a lack of it does often cause stress, worry, anxiety and all sorts of problems. As long as you nurture your soul and focus on happiness first, having money can yield more freedom, choices, and resources to keep yourself or give to those important to you.

When you think of success, is there a monetary value that you attach to this? E.g. that you'll only be successful once you live in a particular style of house, have paid off the mortgage, have material wealth, or earn a certain amount of money?

Or do you limit yourself through your negative beliefs about money?

If any measure of your success relates to the attainment of a financial goal or something that costs money, then it is critical that you develop a positive relationship with money – what you think and feel about having it or not having it! To do this, note the beliefs that you have in relation to money (you could start by filling in the blanks in the statements above) and then use tapping, affirmations or another intervention such as NLP or Hypnotherapy, to turn around any negative associations. And then notice what happens...

Your relationship with success

Your relationship with success is dependent upon what you think and feel about yourself (as I discussed in Principle One), how you define and measure success, and how you feel about failure.

• What do you think and feel about success?

• Are you scared of success?

• Are you scared of failure?

• How will you know when you're successful?

Just recently I was discussing success with a couple of my clients. One client mentioned that she measures success by the attainment goals. However, while she had smashed all her business goals for this year, she still didn't feel successful. When we explored this further, she said it was because she felt she needed to beat her goals on a regular basis. Yet it was only after we'd pointed out she'd been beating her goals for months, that she gradually began to accept she is successful now – she is already the person she'd been seeking to become.

Not that long ago, someone asked me, 'Are you not disappointed that you've not been as successful as you could have been?' Initially I was taken aback by their question, until I realised that their definition of success was so different to mine. For me success is about being happy, healthy, and living a life of meaning with the ability to tap into whatever I need for me to enjoy my life. But for them it was all about getting to the top of the career ladder and having lots of money (despite the fact that they often talked about how unhappy they were). There is no right or wrong, though I do find it really sad that so many people sacrifice their happiness and health in the pursuit of success and material goods, rather than finding it within themselves.

As I shared in Chapter 16, if you want to achieve your goals and enjoy the benefits of success, it's vital to believe your goals are possible, that you have the ability to succeed, and that you deserve to, too! And that's where a detox of your mind to overcome any thoughts and feelings that may be holding you back (including those relating to success and failure) is so important.

Rather than only thinking of success as relating to a material or long-term goal, I'd like to suggest you engage your heart every day so you celebrate the smaller nuggets of success, too. By doing this, you'll have a greater awareness of how successful you already are. You could start by asking yourself the following questions:

• What could I celebrate today?

• How do I choose to feel happy or successful today?

• What progress have I made today?

Your relationship with nature and the planet

We are all pearls in a galactic universe where connection is the key to our survival. You may think of yourself as completely separate to everything else you see around you, but we are, in fact, all connected. At a quantum level we are all part of a greater soup of energy particles.

Without oxygen, water, heat, and light, there would be no planet – you would not exist. Without food you would die. You are a part of nature, whether or not you are someone who enjoys being outdoors. Everything you do and feel has an impact on the environment around you, whether human or otherwise. What you feel not only has an impact on the physical make-up of your body and what you do, but also on others in terms of what they feel, how they are physically, and what they do.

This happens because you are nature, and being outside in a healthy environment is natural – it feeds your body, mind, and soul.

I remember when I was young I didn't think this was important because I hadn't experienced the outdoors as much as inner city living and indoor activities. However, I've since discovered how much more energised I feel when I'm outside. Now being outside and being mindful of my impact on the planet as a temporary inhabitant, has become part of my daily life. Likewise, I cherish the moments I spend time with my cats.

How could you enjoy a better connection with nature or the planet?

In Summary

Relationships are a key component of your happiness and success. They have the capacity to be the glue of society or destructive shards of glass.

You deserve to enjoy happy harmonious relationships but your reality is dependent upon on how you treat yourself and others; how much you invest in or neglect building meaningful relationships; who you spend your time with; your relationship with the environment, and all other facets of life. If you want to enjoy more love, happiness, and success, first decide how to change yourself and take action aligned to what you'd love to experience.

Resourceful Questions

- How could you be more loving, kind, compassionate, respectful, appreciative, or honest with others?

- How could you improve your relationship with XXX?

- What type of relationship(s) would you like to enjoy?

- Which relationships would it be good to improve, or let go of?

Empowering Affirmations

- I love feeling connected to my authentic self.

- I'm so grateful to be surrounded by happy, harmonious and loving relationships.

- I'm ready to attract my ideal partner/friends.

- I have positive associations to money and success.

Tapping 'Set Up' Statements

- Even though I'm not yet sure who I really am, I love and accept myself.

- Even though I'm not happy with my relationship with XXX, I deeply and completely accept myself.

- Even though I avoid 'difficult' conversations, I know I deserve to be heard and be happy.

Recommended Resources

- *Take Flight! Master the DISC Styles to Transform Your Career, Your Relationships...Your Life* by Merrick Rosenberg & Daniel Silvert

- *Nonviolent Communication* by Marshall B. Rosenberg

- *The Five Love Languages* by Gary Chapman

- *Creating Affluence* by Deepak Chopra

- *Rich Dad, Poor Dad* by Robert T. Kiyosaki & Sharon L. Lechter

- *Think & Grow Rich* by Napoleon Hill

- *Money & The Law Of Attraction* by Esther & Jerry Hicks

- *The 7 Graces Of Marketing* by Lynn Serafinn

Chapter 19

Principle 9 – Tap Into Natural Energy Sources For Peak Performance

Nurture, listen and respond to feedback from your heart, mind, body, soul, and universal intelligence for optimum performance, increased energy, longevity, and to attract what is in the highest good of you, others, and the planet.

You'll know yourself, to be happy and successful you need to feel good and have the energy to take effective action towards your goals. That when you're not feeling great, it's more of a struggle to get through the day – you may not achieve all you intend to do in the way you'd like, or be yourself with others.

Many people think they get all their energy from what they eat, what they drink, and by getting sufficient sleep. While eating a healthy diet and sleeping are critical if you want to enjoy life and to perform to the best of your ability, there are other factors that influence the energy you have, too. These include your physical health, how active you are, what you think, how you feel emotionally, how effective you are in managing your emotions, who you spend time around, the Earth's geometric field, and even the weather in space.

When applying the heart values of loving and respecting yourself in the context of your health, you refrain from nurturing unhealthy habits or addictions that will cause you harm. You instead do what it takes to be as fit and healthy as possible. That is what this principle is about – nourishing your mind, body, and soul for success by taking action to put yourself in the best place physically, mentally, emotionally, and spiritually. All these influence your energy levels and your energy vibration – the vibes you give off.

Fuel Your Body for Success

There are a wealth of resources available on what to eat, drink, and how to exercise, so I'm mainly going to focus on the non-physical aspect of your being; sharing how you can tap into the natural energy field you are part of so you can make better choices and decisions to boost your success. Before I do, let me share my top tips for feeding your body for success:

1. Consciously choose what to feed your body – when you hold the intention of loving and respecting your body, it's not so easy to consume harmful food, drink, or toxic substances. Especially if you tap away any cravings or desire for what you know isn't good for you.

2. Master your emotions so you are not tempted to comfort eat, so you feel more motivated to be active and so the chemicals pumping through your body are doing good not long-term harm. Feeling stressed, anxious, scared, angry, hateful or resentful all the time is a sure way to be ill, and increases your chance of a heart attack and premature death.

3. Move as much as possible each day and at least every twenty minutes – a sedentary lifestyle is one of the main contributing factors for heart attacks, strokes, and obesity, many of which could be avoided.

4. Get a food intolerance and allergy test done – it's amazing how many people have intolerances that are causing them to be ill, bloated, lack energy or cause other diseases. I remember wishing I was one of the lucky ones with a flat stomach – only to discover a few years ago, I do have one if I don't eat wheat! And that I don't need to have red blotches on my skin if I stay away from red wine. What you eat has a huge impact on how you feel, what you do, and how long you live.

5. Find some form(s) of exercise that you love – there are so many ways to be active for people of all ages and physical abilities. There are many inspirational stories of those who have achieved all sorts of sporting feats in the face of adversity, including those participating in the Paralympics, and injured war veterans. Check out the Internet for inspiration and local activities you could get involved in.

Other Natural Energy Sources

The chances are that you'll remember the devastating 2004 Boxing Day Tsunami in Asia which tragically claimed the lives of over two hundred thousand people. But did you hear the extraordinary stories about the majority of wildlife that escaped before the Tsunami hit land? Across Asia there were independent reports from wildlife parks and the coastal regions of Sri Lanka, Thailand and India, that few animals died because they'd already fled to safety inland or to higher ground.

Whilst some believe animals have a sixth sense that enables them to avoid impending disaster, there is no scientific evidence that proves this (it isn't easy to replicate this in a lab or 'real' setting). However, there is little doubt that some other species appear to either have more acute senses or are more in tune with nature than humans. For example, many species of birds, turtles, and whales are able to navigate long distances with great accuracy, due to their ability to tap into the earth's magnetic field.

In the case of the Asian Tsunami, local wildlife specialists believe the animals sensed 'waves' of energy from the earthquake that caused the tsunami, and paid attention to subtle differences in atmosphere and environment that humans don't notice or didn't know to treat with alarm, e.g. a receding sea. Whatever the reason, their ability to tap into natural energy sources certainly saved their lives.

Every year elephants travel hundreds of miles along the same paths as their ancestors (other than when they need to go around man-made obstacles). They are also known to experience extreme grief when they lose a member of their family. However, wildlife experts were still surprised by what happened when the author, conservationist and 'Elephant Whisperer' Lawrence Anthony died. Inexplicably, within hours of his death, a couple of herds of elephants (including some he'd rescued) travelled over 12 hours for a two-day 'elephant' vigil at this home. How did they know about his death?

Whether you view these as coincidences, synchronicity, a sixth sense, or something else, it doesn't really matter. There are many events science can't yet explain that will form future research projects. However, the one thing we do know scientifically is that you are part of a greater whole – you are a mass of vibrating energy particles that make up what you see, feel, and think of as your body. Everyone and everything around you is also a mass of vibrating particles, and collectively we make up a highly organised universe that is so predicable scientists have worked out how to land with precision on the moon and to do all sorts of other incredible feats in space.

'A human being is part of the whole, called by us "universe", a part limited in time and space. He experiences himself, his thoughts and feelings as something separated from the rest – a kind of optical delusion of his consciousness.'

Albert Einstein

How would it be if, like animals, you could also tap into a natural energy field, to boost your success in any area of life, to avoid potential danger, or to take your performance to the next level?

As a human being, you are one most evolved species on the planet and science also shows you are an interactive part and co-creator of the natural energy field. A living entity who is constantly transmitting and receiving information.

- Fifteen minutes after the first plane hit the World Trade Center in September 2001, two satellites recorded changes in the Earth's magnetic field, causing scientists to change the way they thought about our relationship with the world we live in.[49]

Subsequent studies by Princeton University and The Institute Of HeartMath found that the magnetic fields produced from heart-based emotions such as gratitude, compassion, and forgiveness, affect others and impact the Earth's magnetic field. [50] In other words, when you choose to feel these emotions, you not only change your emotional state and influence how others around you feel, you are also affecting the world we all live in, too. Isn't that amazing!

- There have since been many other studies that show the affect of engaging in heart-based emotions. In 1973 a study across twenty-four US cities showed that crime rates decreased by an average of sixteen percent when just one percent of the population practised Transcendental Meditation.[51]

- But it is not just the Earth's magnetic field that influences your success and governs rhythmic changes in your body – so, too, do the sun and the planets. They are encased by magnetic fields, and changes in their magnetic

---

49 *Global Coherence Initiative - a collaborative science based project between The Institute of HeartMath and internationally renowned astrophysicist and nuclear scientist Dr Elizabeth Rausher) is building a Global Coherence Monitoring System to measure fluctuations in the magnetic fields. http://www.glcoherence. org/monitoring-system/about-system.html*

50 *Gregg Braden, Consciousness And Intentionally Creating Emotion To Help Heal Yourself And Your World, HorizonsMagazine.com, August 2011, http://horizonsmagazine.com/blog/?p=16149*

51 *The Maharishi Effect: https://www.mum.edu/about-mum/consciousness-based-education/tm-research/ maharishi-effect/*

fields impact the Earth's magnetic field. Which in turn affects all life on Earth and the technology that many of us rely on. Cosmic activity or space weather is constantly happening in our solar system to the extent that geomagnetic storms can result in power failures, disrupt wildlife migration flows, and even trigger an increase in the number of sudden deaths from heart attacks.[52]

• Another interesting body of work is that done by the scientific researcher Dr Masaru Emoto, who discovered that water holds and transmits human feelings. He found that when water is exposed to positive loving words or music, the frozen crystals of the water form beautiful crystals. However, when water is exposed to negative words, the crystals are dull and disfigured. Since learning this, I often write love, peace, or happiness on a bottle of mineral water before drinking it.

Managing Your Energy Vibration

While there are many external factors at play, there is still a lot you can change about your day-to-day experience. Remember, every thought and feeling you have has an energy frequency associated with it, and collectively these make up your energy vibration – the vibes you give off to others. Managing your energy vibration is important because if you don't, you could inadvertently be sending out signals that will attract reactions, people, and situations you don't want.

In the 1970s, psychiatrist and consciousness researcher Dr David Hawkins used Applied Kinesiology and Muscle-Testing to develop a research based 'Map of Consciousness' – one that links different energy frequencies to specific emotions on a scale of 1-1000, and can be used to measure your personal energy.[53] At the lower end of the spectrum are negative emotions such as grief (75), fear (100), and anger (150), while at the higher end you have love (500), joy (520), peace (600), and enlightenment (700-1000). He found that people vibrating at a level lower than 200 were mainly focused on personal survival. Those with energy vibrations above 500 enjoyed more happiness, had greater spiritual awareness, and more concern for others.[54]

52 *The Intention Experiment, Lynne McTaggart, Harper Element, 2008, p144-145.*

53 *Power Vs Force, Dr David R. Hawkins, Hay House, 2002, p68-69*

54 *Power Vs Force, Dr David R. Hawkins, Hay House, 2002,*

Or to put it another way, you're more likely to attract happiness, health, and prosperity when you ooze love or peace.

Dr Hawkins also estimated that the energy vibration of mankind as a whole in the 1990s was 207[55] with 85% of the world's population resonating below 200.

However, the good news is that you can raise your energy vibration. And when you reach 500 or above, you'll not only attract more personal success, you'll also help raise the energy of 750,000 individuals who were below the level of 200. Collectively, the 15% of people above 500 have the capacity to counterbalance the lower vibrations of the rest of the global population.[56] Dr Hawkins explains how to measure your energy vibration using muscle testing in his book *Power Vs. Force*.

Another way of putting yourself in a good energetic state is to 'balance your chakras', the seven energy centres in your body which energy flows through. When any one of these is blocked, this can lead to illness and negative outcomes in the area of life to which that blocked chakra relates. By clearing the blockage, you can return to harmony in your body and attract more positive outcomes as a consequence.

Trusting Your Instincts

On a cold, wet and dark winter evening in December 1998, I was shown round a property that had been presented to me as a good investment opportunity. Being self-employed, the 'sensible' part of me had decided to invest in property as my retirement provision, even though my heart wasn't excited about this wealth-creation strategy.

I remember walking into the flat and feeling it was quite a lot to take on; it needed to be completely gutted and done up, and was an hour or so from where I lived. But even though my instincts were saying 'NO!', my head was telling me that the maths added up. So I bought what became a horrendous and costly refurbishment job, with so many 'hidden' issues that needed attention. Then the property market collapsed, and in just three months I'd lost all the capital I'd invested, and owed more to the bank than the value of the flat.

55 *Power Vs Force, Dr David R. Hawkins, Hay House, 2002, p285*

56 *Power Vs Force, Dr David R. Hawkins, Hay House, 2002, p282*

Had I known then how to tap into my intuitive intelligence before deciding whether to buy, I could have saved myself a lot of money – and many sleepless nights!

Has there ever been a time when you wish you'd trusted your instincts?

Or sensed when something didn't seem 'right' about someone?

Sometimes we don't know why we feel or think a particular way, we just do.

As a human being you have the ability to unconsciously tune in to others' energy and to sense if all is well. You do this through your senses, which pick up cues at a conscious and unconscious level, including the subtleties of body language, the way in which someone talks, changes in the atmosphere, environment, nature, and energy field. It's just that most people have been conditioned to ignore their 'sixth' sense and don't know how to spot the signs.

'Our sixth or psychic sense is not a physical sense like the other five – it's more of a spiritual sense, which is connected to our soul body and centered in the heart.'

Sonia Choquette

There are many ways to develop your intuition, including:

• Learn how to embrace the now and be more present in the moment – e.g. by letting go of thoughts and feelings about the past or future, shifting your focus to what's happening around you, or practicing mindfulness.[57]

• Notice what you feel in your body, and act upon what it tells you – through physical sensations, it will let you know if what you're about to do is in your best interest.

It's worth noting, however, that quality of your discernment is a reflection of your beliefs, memories, and associations stored in your mind and body at any point in time; the more pure these are in terms of being clear of negative thoughts, emotions, and toxic substances, the better your ability will to be able to interpret situations accurately. As you can imagine, if you've got too much snow on your aerial or satellite dish, the picture you get on your TV will be fuzzy.

---

57 *'Mindfulness is an innate capacity of the mind to be aware of the present moment in a non-judgemental way. It promotes a way of being that helps us to take better care of ourselves and lead healthier lives. It also enables us to access inner resources for coping effectively with stress, difficulty and illness.' University Of Aberdeen, http://www.abdn.ac.uk/study/courses/postgraduate/taught/studies_in_mindfulness*

- Speak to your unconscious mind and ask for guidance ahead of making decisions – there are various ways to do this, and the easiest way is to simply ask yourself, 'Is this the best thing for me to do?' Then pay attention to what your mind or body tells you.

- Meditating to quieten your mind and increase your sensory awareness. Meditation is also a great way to reduce stress, improve your physical and mental health, boost your confidence, and help you sleep.

Creating Coincidences

It was on date number three that I decided to tell my now husband about the way I live my life. I knew I liked this gorgeous guy sitting in front of me, and for the first time in years I also had the inner strength to assert that he had to accept the true essence of who I am, and my approach to life, if our relationship was to continue.

I remember explaining to him that I often made decisions based on my intuition and 'signs'. That when I decide I want something to happen, I 'put it out there' and it frequently appears. That in my world there is no such thing as coincidences, but rather a constant flow of synchronicities that we can influence to a great extent. I noticed a look of confusion before he warmly replied, 'I'm not really sure what you mean but I'm OK with that...' His response brought joy to my ears – at least this scientifically-minded engineer wasn't put off!

Later that evening, we were sitting in a bar chatting about how good it would be to get cheap flights from Edinburgh to Barcelona for a weekend away (at a time before they were readily available). I commented that all we needed to do was to 'put it out there' and that if this were an option, we'd soon know about it. Then we moved on to another topic of conversation. A few minutes later, I noticed he was distracted. Gazing past me, he said, 'Is that one of your signs?' I turned in the direction he was looking and saw a bus stopped at traffic lights directly in front of us. Along the side of the bus was an advertisement for flights from Edinburgh to Barcelona for £25.99. 'Yes,' I responded, 'and if you want to continue seeing me, you need to be comfortable with that type of thing happening all the time.'

Rather than leaving moments of synergy and flow to chance, there are ways you can choose to experience them more often.

Have you ever thought about calling someone, only to find they phone you shortly after?

Or sensed that something was about to happen, and it did?

Inviting 'coincidences' or synchronicity to happen is a great way to solve problems with less effort. And often what you're presented with is better than what you'd come up with if you limited yourself to your own thoughts. You also open more doors of opportunity too.

Since being introduced to this concept when reading the *Celestine Prophecy* by James Redfield, making requests to the Universe, paying attention to 'signs', and trusting my instincts have all become core components of the way I now live my life – because I know more opportunities flow and I make better decisions when I do. To ignore 'signs' would be like going on a road trip and ignoring the signposts. Instead, I decide what I'd LOVE to happen, set the intention for the 'right' solution to present itself, notice what happens, and act accordingly.

That's exactly what resulted in me going to Rwanda. I remember when I first saw the film about the work Dr Lori Leyden was doing there, I felt compelled to contact her – to find out more, and how I could support her. Just the previous day I'd walked away from a lucrative training contract that no longer resonated with my values and had set the intention to work with a charity where I could make good use of my skills, support young people, and travel. I was so excited (but not surprised) to get an email about Lori's project in my inbox the very next morning. At first, my head tried to stop me from reaching out to Lori for fear of rejection. Previously I would have given in to these doubts, but this time the feeling of alignment to my purpose and connection in my heart was so strong that I trusted my intuition and hit 'send' on my email. Two days later we had a Skype call, and three months later I was in an orphanage up the top of a mountain in Rwanda. It felt like such an easy and natural decision to make, and was one of the best decisions I've ever made in my life!

If the concept of synchronicity is new to you, I suggest first of all that you record all the 'coincidences' that happen, so you can increase your awareness of any patterns that emerge. Then start to set your intentions for what you'd love to happen and notice what does. When it works, that's great! When it doesn't, that's feedback that you may need to raise your energy vibration first (see below).

The Law of Attraction

Are you attracting what you want or don't want in your life?

Just like the laws of nature facilitate the growth of seeds into beautiful flowers, there is also a natural force that supports you in life. A resource you can tap into to attract more of what you'd love to experience, to minimise your exposure to undesirable events, and to help you cope with life's challenges.

All you need to succeed already exists – either within you, through others, or in the collective field of consciousness.

The Law of Attraction is based upon the principle that 'like attracts like' and through your energy vibration this is what leads you to attract much (though not all) of what you experience in life. It's a natural force that's always in motion, whether or not you're consciously aware of it or choose to activate it.

If you're giving off positive vibes aligned to your goals or desired outcomes, then you're more likely to achieve them. However, transmitting negative vibes – e.g. by giving in to fear, anxiety or nerves – will often attract more of what you don't want. In other words, when you're not getting the results you'd like, that's feedback that there is a misalignment of one of the four elements of Heartatude – your purpose, thoughts, feelings, or actions.

There are obviously some things that you can't control in life that you definitely wouldn't consciously choose to experience. But you do because they are part of life's cycle or for reasons that are not within your control. Some undesirable events may be very traumatic and devastating at the time, but it is possible to heal from most wounds if you want to, and get support to help you to do so. In this book I'm mainly referring to activities which you can control or influence, though depending on your belief system, you may view all that happens to you in this life, the good and the bad, as part of your soul's journey. If this is the case, please do apply what I share in that context.

I used to struggle with manifesting what I wanted, consistently. Over the years I'd read many personal development books and attended numerous courses in my quest for happiness. I'd learned to cope well with most of life's challenges and to be happier than I'd been before. But it took me a while to attract abundant flow of success through my business. I'd mostly enjoyed the transition from a 'successful' but unfulfilling career to running a sustainable business. But there were times when it felt like a struggle too. Particularly as I waded through finding my focus, learning new skills, and overcoming doubts and fears. A lot of the time, I felt frustrated as I did what the 'experts' taught, but didn't get the results I so craved.

I felt I was missing something – as though there was a piece of the puzzle that had got lost in translation. I couldn't understand why what I was doing wasn't working. At the time, I didn't understand the part my emotions, subconscious mind, and energy vibration played in the results I was attracting. While I was 'doing' all the right things, I was still operating from some fear-based thoughts and emotions inside, and that meant I was energetically sending out mixed and unclear messages – to those around me, and to the outer world. The inconsistent blend of messages I was projecting was what had been attracting variable results.

Then one day in January 2012, I got it. I'd taken time out over Christmas to re-evaluate my business and to put myself in a better place to succeed, using many of the techniques I've shared with you in this book. This involved getting clarity on who I was, what I wanted, and how I wanted to be of service to others. Then I set myself a few goals, and did a few things to align my head and heart to my goals (including having a Theta Healing session from a friend).[58] The very next day I awoke feeling as though I'd joined the fast lane of a super highway, completely aligned to the core essence of my truth and with the ability to attract what I wanted in my life far more easily.

Over the next few weeks I noticed that when I chose to feel love, joy, and peace in my heart, I could access the flow of this super highway. And that when I allowed myself to be pulled along by the current of this strong energy force, the opportunities that presented themselves were manifestations of what I hoped would happen, and often in ways that far exceeded my dreams. I realised what I was experiencing was the previously elusive flow of abundance that I'd heard others talking about. For the first time, I recognised that when I truly open my heart to love and put myself in a positive state energetically, I attract more success.

By comparison, when you are disconnected from the true essence of who you are, or act from a place of unnecessary fear, lack, doubt or frustration, you attract more challenging situations, people, and disappointments over the long-term. Fear is a healthy emotion to feel when you need to take action

---

58 *Theta Healing is an energy healing modality that taps into a meditational brainwave frequency and universal intelligence to create physical, mental, emotional and spiritual changes.*

to save your life. But if you give in to it when making less critical decisions, it holds you back and keeps opportunities at bay. Likewise, when you feed feelings of 'I can't be bothered', 'I'm scared' or 'I can't', you make things harder for yourself.

You really are co-creating your existence through your thoughts, feelings, actions, and ultimately your energy vibration. And a great way to work towards goals or overcome challenges is to raise your energy vibration before taking any other action – by doing this you're likely to find far better ideas, solutions, and opportunities present themselves than you could come up with when you're stuck in your head. In other words, before considering what to do, raise your energy vibration for success and then act upon what comes up.

Unlimited Resources and Potential

Just because you can't see something doesn't mean it doesn't exist. Have you ever seen:

• pure electricity?

• all the information flying around in the air, on its way to satellite dishes and aerials so you can watch TV?

• text messages finding their way through the information soup to appear on the 'right' mobile phone?

• the information 'on the Internet' that you access through your computer or mobile devices?

A premise of the Law of Attraction is that there is an energy field that holds all the information you need, that you can tap into.

The concept of an energy field or source isn't new – it's been around in many cultures and religions for thousands of years. Terms often used to describe who or what you can tap into include God, the Universe, the Creator, the Field, the Matrix, Source, Spirit, Chi, Qui, Universal Intelligence or Supermind. There are many practices that all rely upon an energetic or spiritual field of existence, e.g. prayer, Reiki, Theta Healing, mediums, angels, or spirit guides. Even the concept of trusting in fate or believing 'what's meant' assumes there is something greater at play than us as individuals.

Deciding whether to attract endless possibilities and success rather than a lack of them, is a bit like deciding which radio station to listen to. You choose what you want to experience, then you tune in your radio (or body) into the relevant frequency so that you receive the information that's being transmitted through that particular frequency. There are always other stations transmitting information, but you don't pick them up because you're not tuned in to their frequencies. When your energy vibration is love or above, you attract information, resources, and connections that are also at that frequency.

How would you like to enjoy an easier flow of abundance?

What if everything you could ever want or need is already out there, just waiting for you to connect to it?

Tapping into the infinite field of universal intelligence is a bit like downloading helpful resources and information from the Internet, a cloud, or the energy field they access in the film, *The Matrix*.

What I've found when I'm struggling, or not getting the results I want, is that the easiest way to break through this is to raise my energy vibration. Usually by setting my intentions and then doing some tapping or meditation. I nearly always find that things flow much easier after doing this. What I encourage you to do, is to experiment to see how raising your energy vibration makes a difference to you, too.

How to Raise Your Energy Vibration

Ultimately *Heartatude* and The 9 Principles Of Heart-Centered Success are all about raising your energy vibration to one that attracts greater success – by engaging your heart and taking action aligned to your truth. So you and others around you benefit.

All the tools I share in this book will help you do this, because your personal energy or vibration (and therefore what you attract) is greatly dependent upon what you think and feel in any moment. The more aligned your thoughts, feelings, and actions are to your purpose and what you'd like to achieve, the more likely you are to succeed. By purposefully raising your energy vibration and putting yourself into one of the higher energetic states of positive emotions, such as love and peace, you'll make it easier to succeed. By contrast, if you foster feelings or anger, resentment, bitterness, or hatred in any area of your life, these will sabotage and erode your happiness, success, and even physical health.

The secret is to master how you manage your emotions, because what you feel has such a strong influence on what you'll attract (as well as what you'll do). Since your thoughts influence what you feel, it's obviously important to take control of these, too. Here are some of the strategies I've already discussed for feeding your mind, body, and soul for success:

• Choosing thoughts aligned to your desired outcomes, intentions, purpose, and goals.

• Acknowledging and letting go of negative emotions.

• Engaging your heart so you feel love, peace, gratitude or compassion in your heart more often.

• Spending time outside in nature (ideally in places with minimal pollution).

• Being in service to others.

• Meditating.

• Tapping.

Doing any of these will have a positive effect on the chemical make-up of your body – as, of course, does what you physically eat, drink, and consume.

You can either choose to put yourself in the best place to excel in whatever you're doing, or choose to ignore the incredible natural capacity of your body and the Universe of which you are part.

I'm always so impressed to hear Olympians talk about not only their training regimes and diets but also how many refrain from drinking alcohol for months before the big event, so their bodies become the most efficient machines they can for the event. In a similar way, one of my Reiki practitioner friends is vegan, does not drink alcohol, and meditates daily so her body is the purest vessel it can be for the energy she is channelling. Both athletes and my friend prioritise looking after their bodies and energy so they can perform to the best of their abilities.

The next time you are faced with a challenge or set yourself a goal, use any of the tools I've shared in this book (and particularly those I've mentioned above) to raise your energy vibration before deciding what else to do. I've found it's so much easier to solve a problem when you first raise your energy vibration – before thinking about what to do or taking any action relating to the problem.

Taking this to the next level, there is a growing body of science that shows when you specifically put yourself into a state of personal coherence (when you experience the natural flow of harmony and synergy between your heart, brain, and mind), you will naturally activate your heart's intuitive guidance system. The Institute of HeartMath encourages individuals to adopt heart-based living by taking responsibility for their own thoughts and feelings so they are happier and healthier, and through the Global Coherence Initiative[59] is aiming to create more social accord and ultimately world peace. Their Emwave software is a fantastic way to measure your heart/ mind coherence and reduce stress – personally watching on my computer what was happening in my body, in response to what I was thinking and feeling, was mind-blowing!

In his book *The Matrix*, Gregg Braden talks about how he discovered from Tibetan monks that compassion is not only an emotion you can feel in your body, but is also one of the most powerful resources available to you. That 'compassion is both a force in the Universe as well as a human experience'.[60] In other words, when you choose to experience a deep feeling of compassion, you resonate at a high-energy frequency and are better able to tap into the infinite resources of the Universe.

When I started out on my personal development journey, everything I've covered in this chapter was new to me – but I was curious. My interest was aroused further while in Waterstones Bookstore one day. I was standing browsing the shelves when a book literally fell off one off the bookcases and landed at my feet. As I picked it up, I had to laugh to myself – it was SyncroDestiny (harnessing the infinite power of coincidence to create miracles) by Deepak Chopra. That was one of the first times I consciously remember paying attention to what I now call 'signs'. In that moment I realised I'd been limiting the possibilities for me to be happy and to live a more meaningful life. And so I decided to embrace possibility – to do more of what could work, rather than dismissing what I don't understand. Without a doubt, this shift has been a major contributing factor to the deeper sense of peace, contentment, and resilience I now enjoy.

In Summary

You are part of a Universe of abundant resources just waiting for you to tap into them, so you can make life easier for yourself. I encourage you

---

59 *A science-based project that unites people in heart-focused care and intention, to facilitate a shift in global consciousness, from instability and discord to balance, cooperation and enduring peace. http://www. glcoherence.org*

60 *Gregg Braden, The Devine Matrix, Hay House Publishing, 2007, p87.*

to become curious, too, as you navigate your way through life, and not to dismiss ideas just because you don't have experience of them. To experiment and do what resonates and helps you become the person you'd like to be.

You have so much potential to be happy, healthy, and successful – it's simply a matter of choosing how you want this to shape your destiny. You can tap into the infinite power of being part of an energetic universe that holds all the answers and resources you need to succeed. Or you can choose to ignore it.

What do you think or feel will help you most?

Resourceful Questions

• How could I raise my energy vibration today?

• What daily practice could I adopt to raise my energy vibration?

• How could I feel more positive about XXX?

Empowering Affirmations

• I'm good at manifesting coincidences.

• It's great to realise that I don't need to know all the answers.

• I love how raising my energy vibration helps me work out the best way forward.

• I'm getting better at raising my energy vibration every day.

Tapping 'Set Up' Statements

• Even though I seem to attract what I don't want, I deeply and completely accept I always do the best I can.

• Even though I've not managed to succeed at/in XXX yet, I deeply and completely love and accept myself.

• Even though I don't know if raising my energy vibration will work, I'm open to the possibility it will.

Resources

• *SynchroDestiny* by Deepak Chopra (and Chopra Meditations)

• *Power Vs. Force* by Dr David R Hawkins

- *Loving Yourself To Great Health* by Louise Hay, Ahlea Khadro & Heather Dane

- *The Optimum Nutrition Bible* by Patrick Holford

- *Perfect Health* by Deepak Chopra

- The Global Coherence Initiative - http://www.glcoherence.org

- *The Divine Matrix* by Gregg Braden

- *The Field* and *The Intention Experiment* by Lynne McTaggart

- *The Celestine Prophecy* by James Redfield

- *Trust Your Vibes* by Sonia Choquette

- *The Hidden Messages In Water* by Dr Masaru Emoto

- *Destiny Vs Free Will* by Dr David Hamilton

- *The Secret* (book and film) by Rhonda Byrne

- http://www.Loveorabove.com (Christine Marie Sheldon)

- *Choice Point* by Harry Massey and Dr David Hamilton

- Emwave software from the Institute Of HeartMath – http://www.heartmathstore.com

- *The Energy Medicine Kit* by Donna Eden

- *Eastern Body Western Mind* by Anodea Judith

- *Energy Breakthrough Guide* by Christie Marie Sheldon - http://www.loveorabove.com/

PART 3
- Choose Your Future -

Chapter 20

Take Enlightened Action

'We cannot solve our problems with the same thinking we used when we created them.'
Albert Einstein

Miracles frequently unfold when we're in Rwanda, and I'm sure it's because we're less distracted by day-to-day life at home; we're more connected to the love in our hearts by being there with the desire to help, and spending more time tapping, praying, meditating; being surrounded by others who ooze love, compassion, and gratitude, as well as having experienced many miracles beyond their wildest dreams; and because our vision for what we'd like to achieve is so huge. What continually manifests continues to amaze us as we dream big, set intentions, create the resonance of pure love in our hearts, and wait to see what happens!

Developing Your Own Success Formula

One of the keys to success I hope you're taking from this book is to find love and happiness in your heart first, then revolve what you do and aspire to be in life around this. Rather than hoping you'll be happy when you win the lottery, achieve a goal, or experience a milestone in life.

If you attach your happiness to the attainment of something outside you, that's a sure way to keep happiness and contentment at bay. Instead, I encourage you to strive for a more holistic approach to success – one where you focus on feeling love and happiness every day from inside, enjoy personal achievements, bounce back from life's challenges, and make a difference to the lives of others. How does that sound?

I'm not suggesting that's easy, but in my experience once you align your life around the 9 Principles, it's so much easier and rewarding than striving for happiness and success based on others' expectations, not knowing who you are, being bored, depressed or spending too much time aimlessly doing things that make you feel bad! As well as being happier, you may also find you'll have more energy, money and feel less stressed.

What does success mean to you?
What type of success would you like to enjoy?
What do you need to do differently to achieve this?

The 7 Steps to Happiness and Success

In Chapter 2, I shared how aligning your head, heart, and actions to a greater purpose, will help you enjoy the happiness and success that you desire. And that whenever you don't get the result you want (or suffer many physical 'symptoms' of distress), it's because there is a mis-alignment of one of those four factors.

While it can be tempting to stay in your comfort-zone, if you want to feel better or get different results it inevitably requires taking action that is different to what you've done in the past. All through this book I've been sharing tools and techniques you can use to do this. Now I'd like to consolidate all this into a simple process you can apply any time to you'd like to get better results or to feel better.

STOP, turn off your autopilot, and follow these steps, BEFORE taking any other action:

1. **Get clear on your why (PURPOSE)** – why is it important for you to achieve or resolve this? What positive impact do you want to have – on your life, the lives of others, or the planet? How will this make a difference to you? What are the benefits to you and others of achieving this?
2. **Define your desired outcomes (PURPOSE)** – what specifically do you want to experience or achieve in this situation or context?
3. **Be mindful of your positive intentions (HEAD)** – how do you consciously intend to be before, during, and after the event or experience? E.g. to be calm, curious, helpful, confident, fully present, committed, etc.
4. **Focus on what you can control in this situation (HEAD)** – and commit to doing this rather than focussing on what you can't control or influence. This includes what you think (beliefs, and equipping yourself with the relevant skills and knowledge); what you feel (and how you manage

your emotions); and gathering all the necessary resources (e.g. including money, time, and support to help you).

5. **Choose empowering thoughts (HEAD)** – notice what you are thinking about the situation or your goal and replace any negative thoughts with a more positive perspective. As I've already mentioned, you can use a whole range of interventions to change your thoughts, including tapping, affirmations, mantras, NLP, hypnotherapy, Theta Healing or Kinesiology.

6. **Decide how you'd like to feel (HEART)** – notice what you are feeling, take action to let go of any negative emotions, and then to feel the way you'd like to feel, e.g. calm, confident, or at peace. This may involve also learning to love and accept the wonderful person that you are (especially if you don't already feel this). Remember, putting yourself into an emotional state of love, peace, compassion, or gratitude in your heart not only helps you feel good, but it raises your energy vibration for success. Refer to the chapters on 'Engaging Your Heart' or 'Managing Your Emotions' for reminders of how to do this.

7. **Take enlightened ACTION** – once you've aligned your thoughts and feelings to your desired outcomes, take action aligned to these and what you want to achieve or feel. This could include taking practical steps to achieve a goal or it could relate to applying any of the 9 Principles.

Sometimes simply taking the time to pause and contemplate each of these steps ahead of taking action will help you get better results. For more complex situations or goals, you may need to put a lot more in place and to consistently take specific action towards your goal.

Obviously, if you feel you are unable to do this by yourself, please do get the support you need to help you – there are resources available to help most challenges you could possibly ever face in life. So commit to getting it, and start by asking others who may know how.

The Power of Practice

Many people seek instant results or solutions to their problems, but it's your level of commitment, energy, and the action you take that determines your success – especially when you're seeking to create new habits or to learn something new.

People who excel in life are motivated to succeed (they are connected to their 'why' or their 'purpose') and so consistently take action to achieve what they set out to do. Here are a couple of ways you could be purposeful in the action you take:

- If you're working towards a goal, decide what actions you could take each day towards this and commit to doing them. When I'm working towards a goal I usually also have 2-3 small things I'll do each day to build momentum, help keep me focussed, create new habits, and increase the likelihood of me achieving that goal.

- Develop a daily practice that puts you in the best place physically, emotionally, mentally, and spiritually, for success. Most days I take a few minutes to do exercises to strengthen my core (and prevent future back problems), meditate, and get some form of physical exercise. I have other things I do most weeks, e.g. reflecting on successes, challenges I've faced (and how I've overcome them), and setting new goals for the week ahead.

When you practise something again and again, you grow as a person – you permanently extend your comfort-zone. Things that used to feel alien, awkward or clumsy can become something you do unconsciously and may even become new skills or talents.

As well as deciding what you're going to do, it's obviously also important to make sure you create time in your day to do these in a way that doesn't add more stress into your life.

I remember when I first learned a lot of the things I've shared in this book, I was still working in a rigid corporate job and spending a lot of my time each day travelling, so I didn't have much extra time. But when I set my mind to it, I was able to say affirmations and do my 'power dance' in the shower; drink my cup of tea in Starbucks while doing something towards my goals for thirty minutes, instead of being my desk at 7.30am; listening to empowering audios when commuting; or taking a lunch hour to go for a walk. It was only when I became self-employed that I realised *I* was the common denominator in creating the constant 'lack of time' I seemed to regularly face, rather than those I previously 'blamed' at work.

Your Mind/Body Detox

Clearing your mind of mental clutter and your body of emotional triggers is a great way to boost how you feel and open the doors to new opportunities.

Obviously, identifying what could be holding you back is a great place to start. To do this, I suggest you download the Heartatude Questionnaire that's available on my website (see the end of this chapter for details of the link). Completing this will help you decide what it would be beneficial for you to work on first – supported by what I share in this book and from the wealth of other resources available.

Then it's a case of deciding how you're going to commit to becoming the change you'd love to experience in your life, e.g. the daily or weekly practices you will put in place, the support you'll get, or training you'll do to enable you to do this.

If you are familiar with tapping, this could include listing all the limiting beliefs, doubts, fears, and anxieties you have, and to tapping on these to clear them. You can find out more about this in Chapter 15 and Chapter 22.

Manifesting Miracles

Applying all I've shared in this book will help you manifest more of what you'd love to achieve, including many things you may previously have believed were not possible for you. Here are a few extra pointers for tapping into and accessing the endless possibilities:

- Be clear about what you want, and communicate congruent messages in relation to this through your thoughts, feelings, and actions. Remember the power of your subconscious mind – if you consciously say you want to achieve a goal but you're harbouring negative thoughts or emotional triggers in relation to achieving this goal, you're less likely to get the result that you want.

- Your feelings are the language of the Universe at a quantum level, and shape your reality – what you do, how you cope with challenges, whether you will succeed, and what you attract into your world. So engage your heart and learn to spend more of your time feeling higher, resonating emotions, such as love, peace, and compassion.

- Remember what you feel in your heart radiates for up to ten feet around you, so take control of the vibes you are giving off as these affect what you attract back, and have an impact on how others feel and respond around you.

- The Universe (or whatever you want to call the field of collective consciousness) is an obedient servant with unlimited resources – it doesn't know the difference between £1 and £1,000,000 (for you or a charitable

225

cause you support). If you feel uncomfortable about manifesting larger results, and focus on the smaller numbers, bear in mind it's only you who is limiting what you will receive. You could instead tap on feeling good and more confident about dealing with larger numbers.

Your Future is in Your Hands

Today we are living in one of the most exciting times ever. We've access to considerably more resources than previous generations, technology offers the potential to enhance all aspects of our lives, and there's an increasing shift in attitudes from survival of the fittest, to a more compassionate and collaborative approach to success.

Success doesn't have to come at the expense of happiness, others, living a life of meaning, or the planet.

It's hard not to notice the masses around the world coming together, challenging old paradigms – calling for changes in the way we approach every area of life, how businesses operate, how we look after those less fortunate, and how countries are run.

A new global consciousness is emerging, seeking the greater good of all – one that welcomes the coming together of science and ancient wisdom; that respects and cares for all forms of life; that seeks to bring out the best of humanity; and protects the sustainability of the planet.

And at the heart of this is you – like everyone else, you are part of this universe, human evolution, and change. Whether or not you consciously choose to be.

No matter who think you are, you are a unique soul with endless possibilities to live a happy, successful, and rewarding life – and you deserve it! How you choose to feel and what you choose to think and do doesn't just affect you. You are always having an impact on people around you and the world we live in.

So draw upon the strength within you that enabled you to learn to walk (including coping with all the failed attempts), and apply the same determination and practice to creating the life you'd love for yourself. By being the person you were born to be, you are being the greatest gift and support you can be to others.

Imagine a movie being made of your life and the producer filming various scenes; those based on what you say you'd love to happen in your life, and others reflecting what would be likely to happen if you were to make no significant changes today. Then, as happens towards the end of making a film, decisions need to be made as to what scenes to include in the final cut – the scenes that come together to tell the story of your life.

What story would you like a film of your life to tell?

That you grew to become a beacon of light in the world, bringing joy to others? Or that you chose to suffer and wither in darkness instead?

Your future really is up to you!

Commit to Action

It's really powerful to regularly take a few moments to reflect on what you read and to note down any ideas you've had. Remember, if you don't take action, you'll not change how you feel and the results you are getting!

What are your top insights from this book?
How do you feel about what you've read?
What inspired action will you take?

Check out resources to support this book at - www.alisoun.com/heartatude

---

A Few Closing Thoughts

'As more of humanity practises heart-based living it will qualify the 'rite of passage' into the next level of consciousness. Using our heart's intuitive guidance will become common sense – based on practical experience.'
Doc Childre, Founder of The Heart Math Institute

Thank you for taking the time to read this book. Hopefully, it has touched your heart, stimulated thought, and prompted ideas for what you can do to enjoy more happiness, health, meaning, and prosperity in your life.

Living a happy and meaningful life is a wonderful experience I never thought would happen to me. It's not all perfect, there are still things I'd prefer not to be happening and challenging events that still happen. However, I'm so grateful to be equipped with powerful coping strategies and transformational tools that make my dance with life much easier.

Being able to let go of negative emotions such as the sadness, hurt, and disappointment of when my first marriage ended and not having had children, has been one of the most liberating things I've ever experienced. As has building the self-belief and confidence to be myself – that it's more than OK to be different: some people will love me for it, others won't, and that's fine. To me, being anything other than the best we were born to be, is denying not only ourselves but also others of the wonderful unique gift we are.

I also feel truly blessed to be doing the work I do with genocide survivors in Rwanda – without doubt, getting involved in this project has changed me for the better as a person. It's taught me the power of the human spirit to be able to heal itself physically, emotionally, mentally, and spiritually – that when we engage with love and compassion in our hearts, miracles really do happen.

I'd love to hear your thoughts and support you on your journey, so please do connect online (see below for details).

With love and light!

Alisoun x

Let's Connect

If you've enjoyed this book, I invite you to connect on-line. You can find out how at www.alisoun.com/heartatude

---

PART 4

- Resource Kit -

Chapter 21

Affirmations

'I am where I am because I believe in all possibilities.'
Whoopi Goldberg, Actress

Throughout this book I've been sharing 'affirmations' that you can use to help you succeed. In this chapter, I explain the basics about what affirmations are, plus how to create and use them effectively to boost your success.

Every thought you think and word you say is an affirmation or statement that influences how you feel (emotionally and physically), what you do, how others perceive you, and the results you get.

However, in this context an affirmation is a positive statement that articulates your desired outcome as if it was true for you now. It's about how you'd like to feel, or what you'd like to achieve that is articulated in present tense.

The practice of using affirmations involves consistently and consciously choosing to think and say positive words to re-programme your mind. For example, choosing to believe and feel 'I am calm' versus 'I am stressed'; 'I can do this' versus 'I am useless'; or 'I feel good' versus 'I am fat'.

Often, during workshops, I take attendees through a practical exercise that stuns most people when they discover the difference in their physical strength, based only on changing their thinking between the statements 'I am strong' versus 'I am weak'. But what you say to yourself (and out loud) really does change the chemistry in your body and makes a huge difference to your success – particularly when you change the negative thoughts stored in your subconscious mind.

I remember the first time someone suggested that I could change my life by changing my thoughts. Seriously? I'd never considered where my thoughts came from, let alone that I could actually change them! But I did know that what I'd been thinking until that point wasn't helping me feel the inner contentment I yearned for. So I decided to give 'affirmations' a shot – I had nothing to lose.

And I was surprised to find that after only a few weeks of using affirmations, I felt happier and more in control of my life – both at home and at work. I still clearly remember the first time someone commented on how much they thought I'd changed, that they'd seen me go from being someone who usually ran around stressed to someone who was far calmer and in control. That conversation was the moment I 'got' the power of affirmations – it was so liberating to realise that I had indeed changed my day-to-day experience and how others perceived me, simply by changing my thoughts!

While you may perceive a belief as being 'true' because of your life experiences, it's actually your decision to believe these thoughts (albeit often at an unconscious level) that creates your reality. When you believe positive thoughts about yourself, the world around you, and the potential for happiness or success, you put yourself in a better place to experience this. However, the opposite is true if you doubt yourself, or feel you don't deserve to be happy – you instead create fewer moments of perceived success, and don't feel so happy. When you choose to focus on the positives of a challenging situation, you will often be better able to cope with it.

As the queen of affirmations, Louise Hay, says, 'An affirmation is the beginning point. It opens the way to change. In essence you're saying to your subconscious mind, "I am taking responsibility. I am aware that there is something I can do to change".'[61]

Re-programming your mind for happiness and success may require doing a detox of those negative thoughts and emotional triggers in your subconscious mind which are yielding any undesirable outcomes you are experiencing.

How to Re-Programme Your Mind

To re-programme your subconscious mind, you can either use techniques at a conscious level, e.g. using affirmations, concentrating, and being

61 Louise L. Hay, The Power Is Within You, Hay House, 1991, p33

fully present when learning new skills (such as driving), or repeated and consistent action to create new habits. Much of what you know and believe to be true today will have been acquired by doing this. Alternatively, you can use other interventions that tackle the issue at a subconscious level and often create instant and lasting change, e.g. using tapping, Neuro-Linguistic Programming, hypnotherapy, Theta Healing, or kinesiology.

Techniques that tackle the issue directly at a subconscious level may be quicker, but affirmations are a great starting point and a tool you can use for yourself, rather than needing a practitioner to facilitate your transformation. You get quicker results if you also use tapping, and I discuss tapping in the next chapter.

Using Affirmations

The way you use affirmations to overcome negative self-talk is to come up with a positive affirmation (in one of the formats below) to counteract the negative thought. Then you say and repeat this affirmation (out aloud or to yourself) several times a day until you notice a change in how you feel, or that the results you get reflect this affirmation as a new belief. When you automatically feel and act differently, that's an indication that your belief has changed at a subconscious level.

To keep things simple, you could start by using some of the affirmations I list at the end of the previous chapters relating to the 9 Principles of Heart-Centered Success – write down those that resonate with you and say these repeatedly to yourself or out loud throughout each day.

Ideally, you first identify what negative beliefs it would be beneficial for you to work on. This involves being more consciously aware of what you're thinking, saying, feeling, or doing in any moment. For instance, if you hear yourself thinking a negative thought, decide if it would be helpful to replace this with a more positive and empowering one. Likewise, you can do the same when you become conscious of negative comments you say out loud. Remember what I suggested in Chapter 15 – to use your body as a feedback mechanism for recognising when it could be good for you to take action (which includes thinking differently), rather than tolerating negative thoughts and emotions.

If you want to feel more confident about achieving a goal, you could ask yourself what doubts, fears, anxieties, or negative emotions you feel in relation to achieving this goal, and note these down – so you can then create positive affirmations and choose other strategies to support you in reaching your goal.

How to Create Your Own Affirmations

A very simple formula to use is based upon the PAW Process[62] that I shared in Chapter 16. This works particularly well if you don't know what specific thoughts are holding you back (because it is based upon the fact that most doubts fall into one of three categories – possibility, ability, or worthiness).

In its simplest form, you could think of your goal while at the same time saying, 'It's possible I can do it, I deserve it.'

Or you can identify the goal/outcome you'd like to achieve, then identify the key doubt that is holding you back, and use the following formula to come up with specific affirmations to help you achieve your goal:

• It's possible to…

• I can ..../I have the ability to…

• I deserve…

So, for example, if you really want to go on a special holiday but you're unsure how you'll afford it (yet), you could use the following affirmations:

• It's possible to go to Australia for three weeks (I know others do it).

• I have the ability to save the money/earn more money/sell a few things to raise the cash/take on a part-time job/cut back on my spending/learn how to…

• I deserve a good break/to make my dream come true/to enjoy this time visiting relatives.

Another structure of affirmations is the 4Ps model[63] that I learnt from the wonderful Dawn Breslin.

• Personal – make them about you, not others, e.g. using 'I am' and using your own words.

• Positive – focus on your desired outcomes rather than what you don't want. And use positive language.

62 Joseph O'Connor, NLP Workbook, Element HarperCollins Publishers, 2001, p18-19.

63 Author of Zest for Life, published by Hay House – see www.dawnbreslin.com

- Present – write affirmations in present tense (if you write them in the future tense, your desired outcomes will stay in the future).

- Powerful – evoke positive feelings by using empowering words to make them more powerful.

You'll see many of the affirmations I've shared in previous chapters are written in this format.

Ways to Get Great Results from Affirmations

- Write these in your Success Journal (or create a lovely decorative notebook for this purpose) and glance through this each day.

- Create visual affirmation cards – or buy one of the many packs available.

- Read, say, or listen to your affirmations several times a day, especially each morning and night. It doesn't matter if they don't feel 'true' yet (as long as you don't use them to make claims to others). Remember this is a technique to change what you believe to be true – to create a new reality.

- Write your affirmations on 'Post-Its' or small cards and have these pinned around your home (e.g. on your bathroom mirror or fridge door), or where you work (e.g. on your computer), so that you absorb them more often.

- Record an audio of your own voice saying these affirmations, and listen to it regularly.

Just recently I read a great blog post about a guy who was being driven mad by the requirement to key his computer password into his computer several times a day. He decided to create passwords that were affirmations and mantras that he hoped would help him create more happiness in his life (having recently split up from his wife). For the first month he keyed in a password based on forgiving his ex-wife (and felt much better for having done this) then set passwords to support his new goals. He has since created a whole new happier and healthier life for himself supported by these.

How Long Does it Take for Affirmations to Work?

Because affirmations are a technique you practise at a conscious level, it will take time for you to re-programme your mind. Anything from 14-28 days for a basic belief change. If you've been diligent in saying your affirmations and they don't work, it could be because you need to refine how you've worded your affirmations. Or you may need another type of intervention to tackle the root cause at an unconscious level, particularly if what you're trying to overcome is a deep-rooted emotional issue, trauma, phobia, or fear. And this is why using tapping (that is easy to learn and works at a subconscious level), together with affirmations, is such a powerful combination.

The purpose of this chapter is to give you an introduction to affirmations and fortunately, because this is a technique used by so many people, there are lots of resources available both online, in books, and as packs of affirmation cards.

Other Resources

- *You Can Heal Your Life* by Louise Hay
- *Zest For Life* by Dawn Breslin

Chapter 22

Tapping

'Our mind takes an inventory of past events and uses them to project the probability of success in the future. Depending on the information it gathers, we either move forward – or the fear response is triggered and forward progress is circumvented.'

Nick Ortner, Author & Founder of *The Tapping Solution*

At the end of each chapter I've been sharing 'tapping set up statements' for you to use to help you overcome physical, mental or emotional blocks that could be hindering your success.

What is Tapping?

Tapping[64] is an incredibly powerful technique that you can easily learn, to quickly and effectively improve most aspects of your life.

In practical terms, tapping is a bit like acupuncture without needles – by using a couple of fingertips to tap on the meridian points on your body, tapping can help you overcome many physical, emotional, and mental issues. You can use it as a painkiller, to reduce anxiety, banish food cravings, attract more money, lose weight, let go of stress, overcome doubts, fears or phobias, stop smoking, pick yourself up when you're feeling down, and so much more.

The great benefit of tapping is that you can use it any time yourself. And because it works at an unconscious level, you'll often get quick and lasting change (when it's done properly). Mastering tapping and affirmations is a potent combination.

---

64 *The word 'tapping' used to collectively describe a range of similar interventions that include Thought Field Therapy (TFT) and a simplified version of this that is known as Emotional Freedom Technique (EFT).*

It is such a powerful technique that it's been used to help war veterans overcome Post Traumatic Stress Disorder (PTSD) and has been the main tool we've taught the young Rwandan genocide survivors to use to overcome horrors they experienced during and after the genocide. The results have surprised us all, with most of those in our programme no longer showing any signs of the severe PTSD they once did! They still remember what they experienced but don't have the same negative emotional charge attached to those memories.

How Does it Work?

'Tapping is based on the premise that "the cause of all negative emotions is a disruption in the body's energy system".'

Gary Craig, Founder of EFT

When your life is under threat, your body does what it can to help you survive – using a part of your brain called the amygdala, it activates your body's 'fight or flight' response – pumping adrenaline round your body, increasing your heart rate, blood pressure and blood sugar, so you can flee from danger. However, in peaceful countries, most of us are fortunate not to face life-threatening situations every day and we've instead developed the ability to trigger similar physical responses in our bodies when we are stressed. Living in a heightened state of alert and having stress hormones pumping through our body, though, is not good for your health over the long-term, and can cause all sorts of physical illness.

Several Harvard Medical School studies found that stimulating certain acupuncture points results in the amygdala's alert system being deactivated.[65] By tapping on the same meridian points, while also focussing on a specific issue, you are effectively communicating to the brain that all is well. The brain then turns off the stress response and your body can return to a state of calm. This type of intervention actually rewires your brain, i.e. it creates new neuro-pathways so that when you tap, you not only change how you feel in the moment, but you can also prevent future stress responses to the same situation (or memory of it).[66]

---

65 *http://tappingsolutionfoundation.org/wp-content/uploads/2014/05/Acupoint_Stimulation_Research_Review-2.pdf*

66 *http://www.thetappingsolution.com/science-and-research/*

Originally tapping was used to help overcome emotional and mental issues. The results led to its rapid growth in popularity, especially when it was also found to help all sorts of other ailments. It's still early days, however, there is now an increasing body of research that show tapping gets particularly good results.

Two leaders in the field of this research are Dr David Feinstein[67] and Dr Dawson Church.[68] In one study, Dr Church measured the impact tapping had on levels of cortisol in the body relative to traditional talk therapy. Although he was only working with a small sample of 83 people, his results were staggering – those who experienced EFT reduced their cortisol levels by 24-50% whilst those who experienced the traditional talk therapies or no intervention didn't show any significant reduction in cortisol levels.[69]

In the UK, various health boards have been exploring the use of EFT including NHS Forth Valley who ran a clinical trial of EFT for treating trauma.[70]

It's an exciting time for tapping, and all those around the world it could benefit as academic institutions and medical schools embark upon research studies examining its effectiveness. It's anticipated that this research will be pushed forward by health services in both the UK and US, who are exploring whether tapping could be a valuable intervention in the bid to reduce healthcare costs.

How To Tap

There are many different ways to tap, and techniques that help with specific challenges. However, here is an overview of the basic tapping sequence (see below for a link to a short demo film on how to do this, on my website):

1. Identify & Rate Intensity Of Your Negative Feeling / Doubt /Physical Challenge / Issue

   Of Feeling / Condition you want to change. Rate its intensity on a scale of 0 to 10, with ten being the worst it could be. E.g. *I'm feeling stressed at work – at a rating of 9!*

---

67 *http://tappingsolutionfoundation.org/wp-content/uploads/2014/05/Feinstein-The-Science_-Why-Tapping-Works_TWS2014_Workbook.pdf*

68 *http://www.eftuniverse.com/research-and-studies/eft-research*

69 *http://www.thetappingsolution.com/science-and-research/*

70 *http://www.heraldscotland.com/hands-on-treatment-offers-hope-for-victims-of-trauma-1.859029*

2. Breathe

   Take a couple of deep breaths in and out, each for the count of five, and continue to breathe slowly the whole way through the tapping sequence.

3. 'Set Up' Statement

   Using the tips of your index and middle fingers of one hand, tap on the 'karate chop point' of your other hand (the outside part of the hand which you would use to deliver a karate chop), while continuously repeating the problem three times in the following format:

   'Even though I feel xxx/have xxx, I deeply and completely accept myself.' (E.g. 'Even though I'm feeling really stressed about work, I deeply and completely accept myself.')

4. Tapping Sequence

   With your fingertips, tap on following points while saying 'reminder phrase' (*a shortened version of the 'set up statement', e.g. 'feeling stressed about work'*).

   1) Top of Head (TOH) – middle top of head.
   2) Eyebrow (EB) – inner side of eyebrow.
   3) Side of Eye (SE) – outside corner of eye.
   4) Under Eye (UE) – 1 inch below pupil.
   5) Under Nose (UN) – between top of lip and nose.
   6) Chin (CH) – midway between chin and lip.
   7) Collar Bone (CB) – 1 inch down & L/R from u-shape notch at bottom of throat.
   8) Under Arm (UA) – side of body even with nipple (men) on bra strap (women).
   9) Repeat the sequence – twice more from the Top Of The Head (step four). You can change the statement slightly, e.g. 'Even though I still feel stressed about work I...' and 'still feeling stressed about work'

5. Review intensity – notice if it's lower or disappeared...
6. Repeat sequence – as long as is necessary, changing statements to reflect new thoughts, feelings or insights.

It may seem odd and unbelievable, but I encourage you to give it a shot and see what happens. There is the potential this will help you overcome many negative emotions, physical conditions, and limiting beliefs!

If you then want to learn more, check out the resources I share below, or arrange to see a Qualified Practitioner who will be able to take you through the process.

Using Tapping for Success

There are so many ways to use tapping, including:

- Whenever you feel any negative emotion you don't want to feel – e.g. stress, anxiety, depressed, frustrated, angry or upset – give it a shot, and continue using if it helps you feel better.

- To clear any doubts or negative emotions you feel in relation to your goals – so you're more likely to perform well.

- If you're on a diet and want to resist your favourite food – I find tapping while looking at whatever I'm tempted by stops the craving very quickly.

- The Personal Peace Procedure – this a great way to detox your mind so you put yourself in the best place emotionally, physically, mentally, spiritually, and energetically. What you do is:

- List all your issues (e.g. doubts, fears, anxieties, upsets, stresses, worries and other negative triggers/feelings).

- Working through your list, one or two a day, tapping each of them away until you no longer feel or believe them. This is particularly powerful if you work on the bigger or deeper issues, e.g. any of the heart values of self-love, self-compassion, being kind to yourself, respecting yourself, forgiving yourself, and letting go of negative thoughts or feelings about the past.

Obviously, please do get support from a professional if you find this upsetting in any way.

To get the best results, be specific in your 'set up' and 'reminder' statements, e.g. 'I feel really anxious about my interview tomorrow' rather than 'I feel anxious'.

The purpose of this chapter was to give you an introduction into tapping if this is new to you. If you'd like to find out more, check out the resources below:

Other Resources

- *The Tapping Solution* (book) by Nick Ortner

- http://www.thetappingsolution.com/ - great resources and research about tapping.

- *The EFT Manual* by Gary Craig / Dawson Church

- *Attracting Abundance* by Carol Look

- *EFT and Beyond*, Edited by Pamela Bruner & John Bullough

- *The Tapping Solution For Weight Loss & Body Confidence* by Jessica Ortner

---

Watch a Tapping Demo

If you'd like to see how to tap, check out www.alisoun.com/tappingdemo

Enjoy!

Recommended Resources

Books, Films & Reports

You'll find a list of resources I recommend at the end of many chapters.

List of Heartatude Tools

Here is a summary of some of the main tools and practical exercises I've mentioned in this book:

Heart-Centered Success Questionnaire	Chapter 2
The Mirror Technique	Chapter 5
Mind Detox	Chapter 5
Kindness Challenge	Chapter 6
Kindness Blast	Chapter 6
Compassion Meditation	Chapter 7
Perspectives Reflection	Chapter 7
UHT Assertiveness Model	Chapter 9
Personal Gratitude Reflection	Chapter 10
Gratitude Journal	Chapter 10
Heart-felt Gratitude Reflection (Audio)	Chapter 10
The Grace Process	Chapter 11
7 Steps To Becoming The Person You Were Born To Be	Chapter 13
The Holistic SMILE	Chapter 15
The PAW Process	Chapter 16
The 5 Steps To Taking Conscious Action	Chapter 17
The 7 Steps To Happiness & Success	Chapter 20
Mind/Body Detox	Chapter 20
Affirmations	Chapter 21
Tapping	Chapter 22
The Personal Peace Procedure	Chapter 22

Alisoun's Website

(http://www.alisoun.com/heartatude)

Free Resources

- **Download Free Resources** - I've mentioned a few free resources in this book to help you boost your success that you can download from http://www.alisoun.com/heartatude using the **promo code – 91nlwn15**

- **Social Media Updates** – I share tips, insights and resources through various social media platforms. Check out www.alisoun.com/heartatude to find out how to connect online.

Products & Services

I offer a range or products and services to individuals, business owners, workplaces, business networks, and community projects, including:

- **Heartatude Course** – experience more transformational exercises or work with me to boost your success. Check out http://www.alisoun.com/heartatude to find out more.

- **Public Speaking** – I am a popular and inspiring public speaker who talks about a whole range of topics covered in this book, plus other topics relating to bringing love, kindness, and supporting social causes into the way business is done. Check out http://www.alisoun.com to find out more.

- **Holistic Training, Mentoring, Blog & Networking For Heart-Centered Business Owners** – to help you feel good as you grow your business with heart. Check out www.alisoun.com for further details and to sign up for free regular business tips and resources.

- **Workplace Training Courses** – I deliver a range of courses in workplaces, including An Introduction To Heart-Centered Leadership, Personal Leadership & Responsibility, Personal Effectiveness and Pure Happiness. To find out more, contact me via www.alisoun.com/contact

PROMO CODE – 91nlwn15

About the Author

Often described as one of the most authentic, inspiring, and heart-centered souls you can meet, Alisoun runs a thriving training and personal development business and has helped thousands of people to enjoy more happiness and success.

Alisoun is a popular speaker, trainer, coach, business mentor, EFT & NLP practitioner, and hypnotherapist. Alisoun also runs The Heart-Centered Network, regularly does humanitarian work with genocide survivors in Rwanda, and is an avid fundraiser.

Prior to this, Alisoun had a successful 20-year career in the investment industry and is full of gratitude every day for being able to enjoy a more authentic and joyful life – living near a beach just outside Edinburgh, Scotland.

You can find out more at http://www.alisoun.com/about

Lightning Source UK Ltd.
Milton Keynes UK
UKOW07f0706160115

244548UK00002B/32/P